# The 30-minute Acid Reflux Diet Cookbook for Beginners

Enjoy 2000+ Days of Delicious Recipes with 30-day Meal Plan to Combat Gastroesophageal Reflux Disease (GERD) & Laryngopharyngeal Reflux (LPR).

Mary Wilson

# Premium Bonuses for Maximum Benefits of this Cookbook

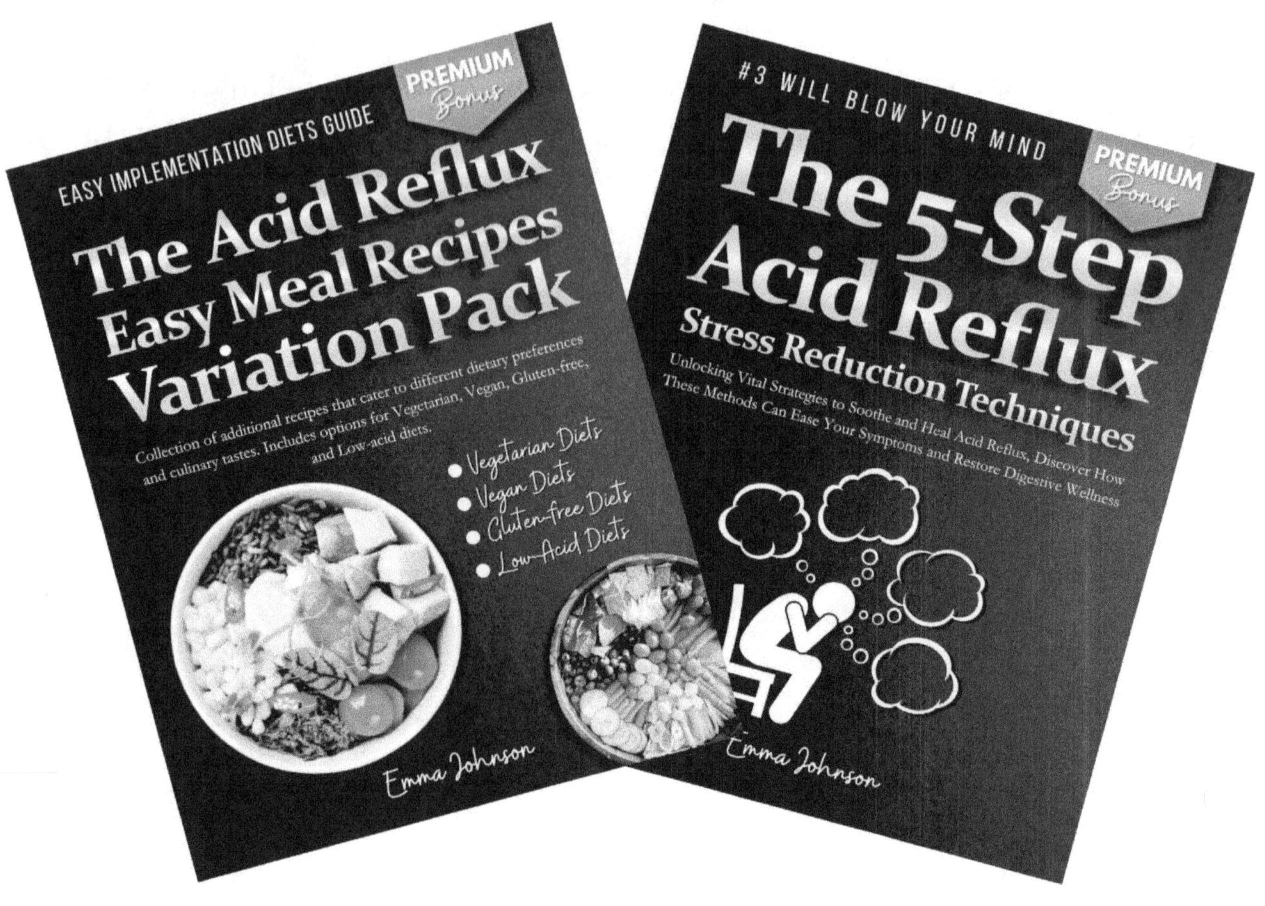


Check the last page of this book to get FREE access
to these premium resources!

# Disclaimer

Please keep in mind that the content in this book is solely for educational purposes. The information offered here is said to be reliable and trustworthy. The author makes no implication or intends to offer any warranty of accuracy for particular individual cases.
Before beginning any diet or lifestyle habits, it is recommended that you contact a knowledgeable practitioner, such as your doctor. This book's material should not be utilized in place of expert counsel or professional guidance.
The author, publisher, and distributor expressly disclaim all liability, loss, damage, or danger incurred by persons who rely on the information in this book, whether directly or indirectly.
All intellectual property rights are retained. This book's information should not be replicated in any way, mechanically, electronically, photocopying, or by any other methods accessible

# Why I Wrote This Book

As I sit down to pen these words, I'm filled with a mix of emotions—reflection, determination, and perhaps a touch of vulnerability. Writing this book, "Acid Reflux Diet Cookbook for Beginners," wasn't just a professional endeavor for me; it was a deeply personal journey born out of my own struggles, experiences, and triumphs in navigating the complexities of acid reflux.

## My Personal Struggle with Acid Reflux

Like many others, my journey with acid reflux began unexpectedly, disrupting the rhythm of my daily life and casting a shadow of discomfort and uncertainty over my well-being. At first, the occasional heartburn and indigestion seemed manageable, dismissed as fleeting inconveniences in the fast-paced rhythm of modern life.

However, as time passed, the symptoms grew more persistent, insidious, and intrusive, encroaching upon the simple joys of eating, socializing, and living fully. The burning sensation in my chest, the discomfort after meals, and the sleepless nights plagued by reflux-induced discomfort became unwelcome companions, overshadowing moments of joy and spontaneity.

I found myself caught in a cycle of discomfort, frustration, and resignation, grappling with the limitations imposed by my body and the relentless persistence of acid reflux. Despite my best efforts to alleviate the symptoms through over-the-counter remedies, dietary adjustments, and lifestyle modifications, relief remained elusive, and the specter of acid reflux loomed large over my daily existence.

## The Turning Point: Embracing Knowledge and Empowerment

Amidst the challenges and setbacks, I found solace and inspiration in the pursuit of knowledge, empowerment, and self-discovery. I delved deep into the vast expanse of research, literature, and personal testimonies surrounding acid reflux, seeking answers, insights, and strategies to reclaim control over my digestive health and well-being.

Through countless hours of research, experimentation, and introspection, I began to unravel the intricate web of factors contributing to my acid reflux symptoms, from dietary triggers and lifestyle habits to stress management and emotional well-being. I learned to listen to my body's signals, honor its needs, and advocate for my own health and vitality with newfound clarity and determination.

Armed with knowledge, resilience, and a growing sense of empowerment, I embarked on a transformative journey towards digestive health and holistic well-being, navigating the complexities of acid reflux with courage, curiosity, and an unwavering commitment to reclaiming my vitality and joy.

**The Birth of a Vision: Sharing Hope and Healing**

As I traversed the winding path towards healing and self-discovery, a profound realization dawned upon me—a realization that would shape the trajectory of my journey and inspire the creation of this book. I realized that my experiences, struggles, and triumphs were not isolated occurrences but shared threads woven into the fabric of a larger narrative—a narrative of hope, resilience, and the transformative power of knowledge and community.

In the quiet moments of reflection, I felt a stirring within my soul—a calling to share my journey, insights, and discoveries with others who may be treading a similar path towards digestive health and well-being. I envisioned a book that would serve as a beacon of light amidst the darkness of uncertainty and confusion, offering practical guidance, empathetic support, and a sense of solidarity to those grappling with the challenges of acid reflux.

I wanted this book to be more than just a collection of recipes and dietary guidelines; I wanted it to be a lifeline—a source of comfort, inspiration, and empowerment for individuals seeking refuge from the storm of acid reflux and reclaiming their rightful place at the helm of their health and vitality.

**The Promise of Hope and Healing**

And so, with a heart brimming with hope and a pen poised with purpose, I set out to embark on the journey of writing this book—a journey fueled by a shared vision of compassion, resilience, and the unwavering belief in the transformative power of knowledge and community.

In the pages that follow, I invite you to join me on a voyage of discovery, healing, and transformation—a journey towards understanding acid reflux, embracing digestive health, and reclaiming the joy of living fully and vibrantly. Together, let us chart a course towards wellness, resilience, and the boundless promise of hope and healing that lies within each of us.

This book is not just a testament to my own journey—it is a testament to the resilience of the human spirit, the power of knowledge, and the enduring promise of hope and healing that unites us all in our shared pursuit of health, vitality, and well-being.
May these words serve as a guiding light on your path towards digestive health and wholeness, illuminating the way forward with compassion, wisdom, and the unwavering promise of a brighter tomorrow.

# Table of Contents

# Chapter 1: Understanding Acid Reflux

Welcome to the journey towards understanding acid reflux and taking control of your digestive health. In this chapter, we will delve into the fundamentals of acid reflux, exploring its definition, symptoms, impact on daily life, debunking myths and misconceptions, emphasizing the importance of diet and lifestyle, and understanding the connection between acid reflux and health.

## What is Acid Reflux?

At its core, acid reflux, also known as gastroesophageal reflux disease (GERD), is a digestive disorder characterized by the backward flow of stomach acid into the esophagus. This phenomenon occurs due to a malfunctioning lower esophageal sphincter (LES), the muscular ring that normally keeps the stomach contents in place.

The LES may weaken or relax abnormally, allowing acidic stomach contents to splash back into the esophagus, leading to irritation, inflammation, and discomfort. This reflux of acid can cause symptoms such as heartburn, regurgitation, chest pain, and difficulty swallowing.

### Recognizing Common Symptoms

Recognizing the symptoms of acid reflux is crucial for early detection and effective management. While symptoms may vary from person to person, common signs of acid reflux include:

- **Heartburn**: A burning sensation in the chest, often after eating or lying down, is one of the hallmark symptoms of acid reflux. It may radiate upwards toward the throat.
- **Regurgitation**: The sensation of acidic stomach contents flowing back into the throat or mouth can cause an unpleasant taste and discomfort.
- **Chest Pain**: Acid reflux can manifest as chest pain, sometimes mimicking symptoms of a heart attack. It's essential to differentiate between the two and seek medical attention if necessary.
- **Difficulty Swallowing**: Known as dysphagia, difficulty swallowing may occur due to inflammation and narrowing of the esophagus caused by chronic acid exposure.
- **Chronic Cough**: Persistent coughing, particularly at night, can be a manifestation of acid reflux irritating the airways.

### Understanding its Impact on Daily Life

The impact of acid reflux extends far beyond physical discomfort, affecting various aspects of daily life. Sleep disturbances, decreased productivity, and avoidance of certain foods and activities are common consequences of unmanaged acid reflux.

Sleep disturbances are particularly significant as acid reflux symptoms tend to worsen at night when lying down. Interrupted sleep patterns can lead to fatigue, irritability, and diminished overall well-being.

The discomfort associated with acid reflux can also interfere with social interactions, work commitments, and leisure activities, diminishing one's quality of life and overall enjoyment.

## Debunking Myths and Misconceptions

In our society, there are numerous myths and misconceptions surrounding acid reflux, contributing to confusion and misinformation. Let's debunk some of the most common myths:

**Myth: Acid reflux only affects older adults.**
Fact: While acid reflux is more common in older adults due to age-related changes in the digestive system, it can affect individuals of all ages, including children and young adults.

**Myth: Acid reflux is merely a nuisance and not a serious medical condition.**
Fact: While occasional acid reflux may be common and manageable with lifestyle modifications, chronic acid reflux (GERD) can lead to complications such as esophageal ulcers, strictures, Barrett's esophagus, and even esophageal cancer if left untreated.

**Myth: Acid reflux is solely caused by spicy or acidic foods.**
Fact: While spicy and acidic foods can exacerbate acid reflux symptoms in some individuals, there are various factors that contribute to its development, including obesity, smoking, alcohol consumption, certain medications, and underlying medical conditions.

**Myth: Acid reflux medications provide a long-term cure.**
Fact: Medications such as proton pump inhibitors (PPIs) and H2 blockers may provide temporary relief by reducing stomach acid production, but they do not address the underlying causes of acid reflux. Long-term use of these medications may also have potential side effects and risks.

By dispelling these myths and providing accurate information, we empower individuals to make informed decisions about their health and seek appropriate treatment and management strategies for acid reflux.

## Emphasizing the Importance of Diet and Lifestyle

Diet and lifestyle play pivotal roles in the management and prevention of acid reflux. Making conscious choices regarding food intake, eating habits, and lifestyle factors can help alleviate symptoms and improve overall well-being.

**Dietary Recommendations:**

- **Avoid Trigger Foods**: Identify and avoid foods and beverages that trigger or worsen acid reflux symptoms, such as spicy foods, citrus fruits, tomatoes, caffeine, chocolate, and fatty or fried foods.

- **Eat Smaller, More Frequent Meals**: Consuming smaller meals throughout the day can help prevent overeating and reduce pressure on the LES, decreasing the likelihood of acid reflux episodes.
- **Stay Hydrated**: Drink plenty of water throughout the day to help dilute stomach acid and promote proper digestion. Avoid carbonated and caffeinated beverages, which can exacerbate acid reflux symptoms.
- **Include Fiber-Rich Foods**: Incorporate fiber-rich foods such as fruits, vegetables, whole grains, and legumes into your diet to promote healthy digestion and prevent constipation, which can worsen acid reflux.

**Lifestyle Modifications:**

- **Maintain a Healthy Weight**: Excess weight, particularly around the abdomen, can put pressure on the stomach and LES, increasing the risk of acid reflux. Aim for a healthy weight through a balanced diet and regular physical activity.
- **Elevate the Head of the Bed**: Elevating the head of the bed by 6 to 8 inches can help prevent nighttime acid reflux by gravity, keeping stomach contents in place while sleeping.
- **Avoid Late-Night Eating**: Allow sufficient time for digestion before lying down or going to bed to reduce the likelihood of acid reflux symptoms at night. Aim to finish meals at least two to three hours before bedtime.
- **Quit Smoking**: Smoking can weaken the LES and increase stomach acid production, exacerbating acid reflux symptoms. Quitting smoking is essential for overall health and can significantly improve acid reflux symptoms.

By making gradual changes to your diet and lifestyle, you can effectively manage acid reflux and improve your quality of life. Remember that small, sustainable changes can yield significant benefits over time.

## The Connection Between Acid Reflux and Health

Beyond its immediate symptoms, acid reflux is intricately linked to broader aspects of health and wellness. Chronic acid reflux has been associated with various complications, including esophageal ulcers, strictures, Barrett's esophagus, and even esophageal cancer in severe cases. Moreover, untreated acid reflux can contribute to poor sleep quality, decreased productivity, and diminished overall well-being. The constant discomfort and disruption caused by acid reflux can take a significant toll on mental and emotional health, leading to anxiety, stress, and depression in some individuals.

Understanding this connection underscores the importance of proactive management and preventive measures. By addressing acid reflux early and adopting healthy lifestyle habits, you can mitigate its impact on your health and well-being in the long term.

In conclusion, understanding acid reflux is the first step towards reclaiming control of your digestive health. By recognizing common symptoms, debunking myths and misconceptions, emphasizing the importance of diet and lifestyle, and understanding the connection between acid reflux and overall health, you can embark on a journey towards improved well-being and vitality.

In the chapters ahead, we will explore practical strategies, delicious recipes, and empowering insights to help you navigate the complexities of acid reflux and embrace a lifestyle of balance and vitality. Welcome to the Acid Reflux Diet Cookbook for Beginners—where every page is a step towards digestive health and wellness.
Remember, you're not alone on this journey. Together, we can overcome the challenges posed by acid reflux and live our best lives.

# Chapter 2: Exploring Longevity and Digestive Health

Welcome to Chapter 2 of our journey towards understanding acid reflux and embracing digestive health. In this chapter, we will delve into the intricate relationship between longevity and digestive well-being, uncover the complexities of the reflux puzzle, shed light on respiratory reflux, explore the link between diet and acid reflux, inspire hope by discussing the reversibility of acid reflux, and finally, embrace the adoption of healthy eating habits for optimal digestive health.

## Exploring Longevity and Digestive Health

Longevity, the pursuit of a long and fulfilling life, is intricately linked to digestive health. The digestive system plays a crucial role in nutrient absorption, energy production, and waste elimination, all of which are essential for overall well-being and longevity.

Numerous studies have highlighted the profound impact of digestive health on longevity. A healthy digestive system ensures efficient nutrient absorption, supports immune function, and maintains a balanced microbiota, all of which contribute to enhanced resilience against disease and aging.

However, the modern lifestyle, characterized by poor dietary choices, sedentary behavior, and chronic stress, has taken a toll on digestive health. The prevalence of digestive disorders, including acid reflux, has risen sharply in recent years, underscoring the importance of proactive measures to promote digestive wellness and longevity.

## Unveiling the Reflux Puzzle

Acid reflux, often described as a puzzle due to its multifaceted nature, presents a complex interplay of physiological, dietary, and lifestyle factors. Understanding the reflux puzzle involves unraveling the mechanisms underlying acid reflux, identifying predisposing factors, and exploring effective management strategies.

The lower esophageal sphincter (LES), a muscular ring located at the junction of the esophagus and stomach, plays a critical role in preventing the backflow of stomach acid into the esophagus. Dysfunction of the LES, caused by factors such as obesity, hiatal hernia, and certain medications, can contribute to the development of acid reflux.

In addition to structural abnormalities, dietary and lifestyle factors play significant roles in exacerbating or alleviating acid reflux symptoms. Consumption of trigger foods such as spicy, acidic, and fatty foods, along with excessive alcohol intake and smoking, can increase the risk of acid reflux episodes.

Effective management of acid reflux involves addressing both the underlying causes and triggering factors. By adopting a holistic approach that incorporates dietary modifications, lifestyle changes, and targeted therapies, individuals can gain control over their reflux puzzle and achieve lasting relief from symptoms.

## Shedding Light on Respiratory Reflux

Respiratory reflux, a lesser-known manifestation of acid reflux, occurs when stomach acid travels beyond the esophagus and reaches the respiratory tract. This phenomenon can lead to symptoms such as chronic cough, hoarseness, asthma, and recurrent pneumonia.
The link between acid reflux and respiratory symptoms highlights the interconnectedness of the digestive and respiratory systems. Aspiration of stomach acid into the lungs can trigger inflammation, irritation, and constriction of the airways, exacerbating respiratory conditions and compromising lung function.

Managing respiratory reflux involves addressing underlying acid reflux symptoms and implementing strategies to reduce the risk of aspiration. Elevating the head of the bed, avoiding late-night meals, and using medications to suppress stomach acid production can help alleviate respiratory symptoms and improve lung health.

## Identifying the Link Between Diet and Acid Reflux

Diet plays a pivotal role in the development and management of acid reflux. Certain foods and beverages can trigger or exacerbate acid reflux symptoms, while others may help alleviate discomfort and promote digestive wellness.
Understanding the link between diet and acid reflux involves identifying trigger foods and making informed dietary choices. Spicy foods, citrus fruits, tomatoes, caffeine, chocolate, and fatty or fried foods are common culprits that can worsen acid reflux symptoms and should be consumed in moderation.
On the other hand, incorporating alkaline-rich foods such as fruits, vegetables, whole grains, and lean proteins can help neutralize stomach acid and reduce the risk of reflux episodes. Fiber-rich foods promote satiety, regulate digestion, and support overall gastrointestinal health, making them valuable additions to a reflux-friendly diet.

## Inspiring Hope: Reversibility of Acid Reflux

Contrary to popular belief, acid reflux is not necessarily a lifelong condition. With the right combination of dietary and lifestyle modifications, along with targeted medical interventions, many individuals can achieve significant improvement in their acid reflux symptoms and even experience complete resolution of the condition.
The reversibility of acid reflux offers hope and encouragement to those struggling with the burden of digestive discomfort. By embracing a proactive approach to health and adopting sustainable habits, individuals can reclaim control over their digestive wellness and enjoy a higher quality of life free from the constraints of acid reflux.

## Embracing Healthy Eating Habits

At the heart of digestive wellness lies a commitment to healthy eating habits that nourish the body, support optimal digestion, and promote overall well-being. Embracing healthy eating habits involves making mindful choices about food selection, portion sizes, meal timing, and eating environment.

Key principles of healthy eating for acid reflux management include:

- **Balanced Nutrition**: Prioritize nutrient-dense foods that provide essential vitamins, minerals, and antioxidants while minimizing empty calories and processed ingredients.
- **Portion Control**: Practice mindful eating and listen to your body's hunger and fullness cues to avoid overeating and minimize pressure on the LES.
- **Meal Timing**: Allow sufficient time for digestion between meals and avoid late-night snacking to reduce the risk of nocturnal reflux episodes.
- **Hydration**: Stay adequately hydrated throughout the day by drinking water and herbal teas to support digestive function and promote overall hydration.
- **Stress Management**: Incorporate stress-reducing techniques such as mindfulness, deep breathing, yoga, and meditation into your daily routine to mitigate the impact of stress on digestive health.

By embracing healthy eating habits as part of a balanced lifestyle, individuals can nourish their bodies, support optimal digestion, and lay the foundation for long-term digestive wellness and vitality.

In conclusion, exploring longevity and digestive health involves unraveling the complexities of acid reflux, shedding light on respiratory reflux, understanding the link between diet and acid reflux, inspiring hope through the reversibility of acid reflux, and embracing healthy eating habits for optimal well-being.

As we continue our journey towards digestive wellness, remember that every step forward is a testament to your commitment to health and vitality. By making informed choices and cultivating healthy habits, you empower yourself to live a life of balance, resilience, and longevity.

In the chapters ahead, we will delve deeper into practical strategies, delicious recipes, and empowering insights to help you navigate the complexities of acid reflux and embrace a lifestyle of balance and vitality. Welcome to the Acid Reflux Diet Cookbook for Beginners—where every page is a step towards digestive health and wellness.

Together, let us embark on this journey towards optimal well-being, one mindful choice at a time.

# Chapter 3: Overcoming Food Addiction and Temptations

Welcome to Chapter 3 of our journey towards understanding acid reflux and embracing digestive health. In this chapter, we will explore the challenges of overcoming food addiction and temptations, emphasize the benefits of incorporating lean, clean, green, and alkaline foods into your diet, discover the role of sugar in acid reflux, promote a balanced and nourishing diet, encourage positive changes in eating habits, and provide insights into the stages of acid reflux.

## Overcoming Food Addiction and Temptations

Food addiction is a complex phenomenon characterized by compulsive consumption of certain foods, often despite negative consequences to health and well-being. Like other forms of addiction, food addiction can have profound psychological, physiological, and emotional implications, making it challenging to break free from unhealthy eating patterns.
Understanding the psychological underpinnings of food addiction is essential for developing effective strategies to overcome temptations and cultivate healthier eating habits. Many factors contribute to food addiction, including biological predispositions, environmental influences, emotional triggers, and learned behaviors.

**Biological Factors**: Certain foods, particularly those high in sugar, fat, and salt, can trigger reward pathways in the brain, leading to feelings of pleasure and satisfaction. Over time, repeated exposure to these foods can lead to tolerance, dependence, and cravings, contributing to addictive eating behaviors.

**Environmental Influences**: Environmental factors such as easy access to processed foods, ubiquitous food advertising, social norms, and cultural influences can shape eating behaviors and reinforce addictive tendencies. The prevalence of fast food establishments, convenience stores, and vending machines makes unhealthy food options readily available and difficult to resist.

**Emotional Triggers**: Emotional factors such as stress, anxiety, depression, loneliness, boredom, and trauma can drive emotional eating behaviors, providing temporary relief from negative emotions and serving as a coping mechanism. Food becomes a source of comfort, distraction, and pleasure, leading to compulsive overeating in response to emotional distress.

**Learned Behaviors**: Learned behaviors acquired through childhood experiences, family dynamics, social interactions, and past traumas can influence food preferences, eating habits, and attitudes towards food. Negative associations with food, such as food shaming or restrictive dieting, can perpetuate unhealthy relationships with food and contribute to food addiction.

## Emphasizing the Benefits of Lean, Clean, Green, and Alkaline Foods

Incorporating lean, clean, green, and alkaline foods into your diet offers numerous benefits for digestive health, overall well-being, and acid reflux management. These nutrient-dense foods are rich in vitamins, minerals, antioxidants, fiber, and phytonutrients, which support optimal digestion, promote alkalinity, and reduce inflammation in the body.

**Lean Proteins**: Lean proteins such as poultry, fish, tofu, legumes, and eggs are excellent sources of high-quality protein, essential amino acids, and nutrients necessary for tissue repair, muscle growth, and immune function. Including lean proteins in your diet can help stabilize blood sugar levels, promote satiety, and support healthy weight management.

**Clean Foods**: Clean foods are minimally processed, whole foods that are free from artificial additives, preservatives, and chemicals. Examples include fruits, vegetables, whole grains, nuts, seeds, and organic dairy products. Clean foods provide essential nutrients, fiber, and hydration, while promoting detoxification and elimination of toxins from the body.

**Green Vegetables**: Green vegetables such as spinach, kale, broccoli, Brussels sprouts, and Swiss chard are nutritional powerhouses rich in vitamins, minerals, antioxidants, and phytochemicals. Green vegetables support digestive health, alkalize the body, reduce inflammation, and promote detoxification, making them essential components of a reflux-friendly diet.

**Alkaline Foods**: Alkaline foods such as leafy greens, cruciferous vegetables, citrus fruits, and almonds help maintain the body's pH balance and counteract acidity, which is beneficial for acid reflux management. Alkaline foods promote alkalinity in the body, reduce inflammation, and support overall health and vitality.

Incorporating a variety of lean, clean, green, and alkaline foods into your diet can help optimize digestion, reduce acidity, and alleviate acid reflux symptoms. By prioritizing nutrient-dense foods and minimizing processed and inflammatory foods, you can nourish your body, support digestive wellness, and enhance overall vitality.

## <u>Discovering the Role of Sugar in Acid Reflux</u>

Sugar plays a significant role in the development and exacerbation of acid reflux symptoms. Excessive consumption of sugar, particularly refined sugars and high-fructose corn syrup, can contribute to digestive distress, inflammation, and acidity in the body, worsening acid reflux symptoms and compromising digestive health.

**Refined Sugars**: Refined sugars such as white sugar, brown sugar, and powdered sugar are highly processed and devoid of nutrients, providing empty calories and spiking blood sugar levels. Excessive consumption of refined sugars can disrupt blood sugar regulation, promote inflammation, and contribute to weight gain and insulin resistance, all of which increase the risk of acid reflux.

**High-Fructose Corn Syrup (HFCS)**: High-fructose corn syrup is a common sweetener used in processed foods, soft drinks, desserts, and condiments. HFCS has been linked to metabolic disorders, liver dysfunction, and increased acidity in the body, which can exacerbate acid reflux symptoms and compromise digestive health.

**Natural Sugars**: While natural sugars found in fruits, vegetables, and dairy products are less processed and contain beneficial nutrients such as fiber, vitamins, and minerals, they should still be consumed in moderation, especially for individuals with acid reflux. Some fruits, such as citrus fruits and tomatoes, may be acidic and trigger reflux symptoms in susceptible individuals.

## Promoting a Balanced and Nourishing Diet

Promoting a balanced and nourishing diet is essential for supporting digestive health, managing acid reflux, and promoting overall well-being. A balanced diet includes a variety of nutrient-dense foods from all food groups, including fruits, vegetables, whole grains, lean proteins, and healthy fats, while minimizing processed foods, refined sugars, and artificial additives.

**Fruits and Vegetables**: Fruits and vegetables are rich in vitamins, minerals, antioxidants, and fiber, which support digestive function, reduce inflammation, and promote overall health. Aim to include a colorful variety of fruits and vegetables in your diet to maximize nutrient intake and support digestive wellness.

**Whole Grains**: Whole grains such as oats, quinoa, brown rice, barley, and whole wheat provide complex carbohydrates, fiber, and essential nutrients that promote satiety, stabilize blood sugar levels, and support digestive health. Choose whole grains over refined grains to maximize nutritional value and support optimal digestion.

**Lean Proteins**: Lean proteins such as poultry, fish, tofu, legumes, and eggs provide essential amino acids necessary for tissue repair, muscle growth, and immune function. Including lean proteins in your diet helps stabilize blood sugar levels, promote satiety, and support healthy weight management.

**Healthy Fats**: Healthy fats such as avocados, nuts, seeds, olive oil, and fatty fish are essential for brain health, hormone production, and absorption of fat-soluble vitamins. Incorporating healthy fats into your diet helps maintain satiety, regulate blood sugar levels, and support digestive function.

**Hydration**: Adequate hydration is essential for optimal digestion, nutrient absorption, and waste elimination. Drink plenty of water throughout the day to stay hydrated and support digestive wellness. Herbal teas, coconut water, and infused water can also contribute to hydration and promote digestive health.

## Encouraging Positive Changes in Eating Habits

Encouraging positive changes in eating habits involves adopting mindful eating practices, practicing portion control, honoring hunger and fullness cues, and cultivating a healthy relationship with food. By becoming more mindful of your eating habits and making conscious choices about food selection, preparation, and consumption, you can promote digestive wellness and enhance overall well-being.

**Mindful Eating**: Mindful eating involves paying attention to the sensory experiences of eating, including taste, texture, aroma, and satisfaction. Slow down, savor each bite, and listen to your body's hunger and fullness cues to prevent overeating and promote digestive satisfaction.

**Portion Control**: Practice portion control by using smaller plates, bowls, and utensils, and being mindful of portion sizes when serving meals. Aim to fill half of your plate with fruits and vegetables, one-quarter with lean protein, and one-quarter with whole grains or healthy fats to create balanced and satisfying meals.

**Honoring Hunger and Fullness**: Tune into your body's hunger and fullness signals and eat in response to physiological cues rather than emotional triggers or external influences. Eat when you're hungry and stop when you're satisfied, allowing your body to regulate food intake naturally and maintain optimal energy levels throughout the day.

**Cultivating a Healthy Relationship with Food**: Cultivate a positive and compassionate attitude towards food and your body, free from guilt, shame, or judgment. Focus on nourishing your body with wholesome, nourishing foods that support your health and well-being, rather than restricting or depriving yourself of certain foods.

By incorporating these positive changes into your eating habits, you can foster a healthier relationship with food, support digestive wellness, and enhance overall vitality. Remember that small, sustainable changes over time can lead to significant improvements in your health and well-being.

## Understanding the Stages of Acid Reflux

Acid reflux is a progressive condition that evolves through various stages, each characterized by distinct symptoms, severity, and implications for digestive health. Understanding the stages of acid reflux is essential for early detection, effective management, and prevention of complications.

**Stage 1: Occasional Symptoms**: In the early stages of acid reflux, individuals may experience occasional symptoms such as heartburn, regurgitation, and chest pain, particularly after meals or lying down. Symptoms may be mild and infrequent, often overlooked or attributed to dietary indiscretions or temporary discomfort.

**Stage 2: Frequent Symptoms**: As acid reflux progresses, symptoms become more frequent and persistent, occurring multiple times per week or even daily. Individuals may experience worsening heartburn, regurgitation, chest pain, and difficulty swallowing, interfering with daily activities and quality of life.

**Stage 3: Chronic Symptoms**: In advanced stages of acid reflux, symptoms become chronic and severe, significantly impacting daily functioning and well-being. Chronic acid reflux may lead to complications such as esophageal ulcers, strictures, Barrett's esophagus, and respiratory issues, requiring medical intervention and intensive management.

**Stage 4: Complications and Decompensation**: In severe cases, untreated acid reflux can lead to complications such as esophageal ulcers, strictures, Barrett's esophagus, and even esophageal cancer. Complications may result in decompensation of digestive function, compromised quality of life, and increased risk of morbidity and mortality.

Understanding the stages of acid reflux allows healthcare providers to assess disease progression, tailor treatment approaches, and implement preventive measures to mitigate the risk of complications. Early detection and intervention are critical for optimizing outcomes and improving long-term prognosis in individuals with acid reflux.

In conclusion, overcoming food addiction and temptations, emphasizing the benefits of lean, clean, green, and alkaline foods, discovering the role of sugar in acid reflux, promoting a balanced and nourishing diet, encouraging positive changes in eating habits, and understanding the stages of acid reflux are essential components of effective acid reflux management and digestive wellness.

By adopting mindful eating practices, making informed dietary choices, and prioritizing digestive health, you can reclaim control over your digestive wellness and embrace a lifestyle of balance, vitality, and longevity. In the chapters ahead, we will delve deeper into practical strategies, delicious recipes, and empowering insights to help you navigate the complexities of acid reflux and cultivate a life of digestive wellness and well-being.

Together, let us embark on this journey towards optimal digestive health and vitality, one positive change at a time.

# Chapter 4: Navigating the Progression of Acid Reflux

Welcome to Chapter 4 of our journey towards understanding acid reflux and embracing digestive health. In this chapter, we will explore the progression of acid reflux, including its stages, complications, and potential treatment options. We will also discuss the importance of seeking professional guidance, empowering yourself through knowledge, and embarking on the acid reflux detox journey for optimal digestive wellness.

## Navigating the Progression of Acid Reflux

Acid reflux is a common digestive disorder characterized by the backward flow of stomach acid into the esophagus, leading to symptoms such as heartburn, regurgitation, and chest pain. The progression of acid reflux varies from person to person and can evolve through different stages, each with its own set of symptoms, severity, and implications for digestive health.

**Stage 1: Occasional Symptoms**: In the early stages of acid reflux, individuals may experience occasional symptoms such as heartburn, regurgitation, and chest pain, particularly after meals or lying down. Symptoms may be mild and infrequent, often overlooked or attributed to dietary indiscretions or temporary discomfort.

**Stage 2: Frequent Symptoms**: As acid reflux progresses, symptoms become more frequent and persistent, occurring multiple times per week or even daily. Individuals may experience worsening heartburn, regurgitation, chest pain, and difficulty swallowing, interfering with daily activities and quality of life.

**Stage 3: Chronic Symptoms**: In advanced stages of acid reflux, symptoms become chronic and severe, significantly impacting daily functioning and well-being. Chronic acid reflux may lead to complications such as esophageal ulcers, strictures, Barrett's esophagus, and respiratory issues, requiring medical intervention and intensive management.

**Stage 4: Complications and Decompensation**: In severe cases, untreated acid reflux can lead to complications such as esophageal ulcers, strictures, Barrett's esophagus, and even esophageal cancer. Complications may result in decompensation of digestive function, compromised quality of life, and increased risk of morbidity and mortality.
Understanding the progression of acid reflux allows healthcare providers to assess disease severity, tailor treatment approaches, and implement preventive measures to mitigate the risk of complications. Early detection and intervention are critical for optimizing outcomes and improving long-term prognosis in individuals with acid reflux.

## Exploring Complications and Decompensation

Complications of acid reflux can have serious implications for digestive health, quality of life, and overall well-being. Chronic acid reflux may lead to a range of complications, including:

**Esophageal Ulcers**: Chronic exposure to stomach acid can erode the lining of the esophagus, leading to the formation of ulcers. Esophageal ulcers may cause pain, difficulty swallowing, and bleeding, requiring medical intervention to promote healing and prevent further damage.

**Esophageal Strictures**: Scar tissue formation in the esophagus can result in narrowing or strictures, making it difficult for food to pass through the esophagus. Esophageal strictures may cause dysphagia, or difficulty swallowing, leading to nutritional deficiencies and impaired quality of life.

**Barrett's Esophagus**: Barrett's esophagus is a precancerous condition characterized by changes in the cells lining the lower esophagus. Individuals with Barrett's esophagus have an increased risk of developing esophageal adenocarcinoma, a type of cancer, highlighting the importance of regular monitoring and early intervention.

**Respiratory Complications**: Chronic acid reflux can lead to respiratory complications such as asthma, chronic cough, and recurrent pneumonia. Aspiration of stomach acid into the lungs can irritate the airways, trigger inflammation, and compromise respiratory function, exacerbating existing respiratory conditions and increasing the risk of respiratory infections.

## <u>Evaluating Medical and Surgical Treatment Options</u>

Medical and surgical treatment options are available for individuals with acid reflux, depending on the severity of symptoms, underlying causes, and treatment goals. Common treatment modalities include:

**Medications**: Medications such as proton pump inhibitors (PPIs), H2 blockers, and antacids are commonly prescribed to reduce stomach acid production, alleviate symptoms, and promote healing of esophageal tissue. These medications can provide short-term relief from acid reflux symptoms but may have side effects and long-term implications for digestive health.

**Lifestyle Modifications**: Lifestyle modifications play a crucial role in managing acid reflux and reducing symptom severity. Recommendations may include dietary changes, weight loss, elevating the head of the bed, avoiding late-night meals, quitting smoking, and reducing alcohol consumption. Lifestyle modifications can help alleviate symptoms and improve quality of life in individuals with acid reflux.

**Surgical Interventions**: In cases where medication and lifestyle modifications are ineffective or contraindicated, surgical interventions such as fundoplication may be considered. Fundoplication involves wrapping the upper portion of the stomach around the lower esophagus to reinforce the lower esophageal sphincter and prevent acid reflux. Surgical interventions are typically reserved for individuals with severe or refractory acid reflux symptoms and complications.

**Endoscopic Procedures**: Endoscopic procedures such as endoscopic mucosal resection (EMR) and radiofrequency ablation (RFA) may be used to treat precancerous lesions associated with Barrett's esophagus. These minimally invasive techniques help remove abnormal tissue and reduce the risk of esophageal cancer in high-risk individuals.

## When to Seek Professional Guidance: Signs and Symptoms

Knowing when to seek professional guidance for acid reflux symptoms is essential for timely diagnosis, appropriate treatment, and prevention of complications. Common signs and symptoms that warrant medical evaluation include:

- Frequent or persistent heartburn
- Regurgitation of stomach contents
- Difficulty swallowing (dysphagia)
- Chest pain or discomfort
- Chronic cough or hoarseness
- Unexplained weight loss
- Blood in vomit or stool

If you experience any of these symptoms, it is important to consult with a healthcare provider for further evaluation and management. Early intervention can help identify underlying causes, alleviate symptoms, and prevent progression to more serious complications.

## Fostering Empowerment Through Knowledge

Empowering yourself with knowledge about acid reflux, its causes, symptoms, treatment options, and preventive measures is key to taking control of your digestive health and well-being. By educating yourself and staying informed about the latest advancements in acid reflux management, you can make informed decisions about your health and advocate for personalized treatment approaches that align with your goals and preferences.
Seek reliable sources of information, consult with healthcare professionals, and engage in open and honest discussions about your concerns, symptoms, and treatment options. Remember that you are the captain of your health journey, and by actively participating in your care, you can optimize outcomes and improve quality of life.

## Embarking on the Acid Reflux Detox Journey

Embarking on the acid reflux detox journey involves adopting a holistic approach to digestive wellness, addressing underlying causes, and implementing targeted strategies to alleviate symptoms and promote healing. Key principles of the acid reflux detox journey include:

- **Dietary Modifications**: Identify trigger foods that exacerbate acid reflux symptoms and eliminate or minimize them from your diet. Focus on incorporating alkaline-rich foods, lean proteins, whole grains, fruits, and vegetables that support digestive health and reduce acidity in the body.

- **Lifestyle Changes**: Implement lifestyle changes such as weight loss, stress reduction, smoking cessation, and regular exercise to optimize digestive function and reduce the risk of acid reflux episodes. Prioritize self-care practices that promote relaxation, mindfulness, and emotional well-being.

- **Supplementation**: Consider incorporating supplements such as digestive enzymes, probiotics, and herbal remedies that support digestive health, alleviate inflammation, and promote gut integrity. Consult with a healthcare provider or registered dietitian to determine the appropriate supplementation regimen for your individual needs.

- **Stress Management**: Practice stress management techniques such as deep breathing, meditation, yoga, and mindfulness to reduce stress levels, promote relaxation, and alleviate tension in the body. Chronic stress can exacerbate acid reflux symptoms and compromise digestive function, highlighting the importance of stress reduction strategies in acid reflux management.

- **Sleep Hygiene**: Prioritize good sleep hygiene practices such as maintaining a consistent sleep schedule, creating a relaxing bedtime routine, and optimizing sleep environment to promote restful and rejuvenating sleep. Adequate sleep is essential for digestive health, immune function, and overall well-being.

By incorporating these principles into your daily routine, you can support digestive wellness, reduce symptoms of acid reflux, and embark on a journey towards optimal health and vitality. Remember that the acid reflux detox journey is a gradual process that requires commitment, patience, and persistence. Be kind to yourself, celebrate progress, and embrace the transformative power of lifestyle interventions on your digestive health and well-being.

In conclusion, navigating the progression of acid reflux, exploring complications and decompensation, evaluating medical and surgical treatment options, knowing when to seek professional guidance, fostering empowerment through knowledge, and embarking on the acid reflux detox journey are essential components of effective acid reflux management and digestive wellness.

By understanding the complexities of acid reflux, advocating for personalized treatment approaches, and embracing holistic strategies for digestive health, you can reclaim control over your health and embrace a life of balance, vitality, and well-being. In the chapters ahead, we will delve deeper into practical strategies, empowering insights, and delicious recipes to help you thrive on your journey towards optimal digestive health and vitality.

Together, let us navigate the path towards digestive wellness and embrace the transformative power of self-care, knowledge, and empowerment in reclaiming our health and vitality.

# Chapter 5: Designing a Two-Week Detox Plan

Welcome to Chapter 5 of our journey towards understanding acid reflux and embracing digestive health. In this chapter, we will explore the process of designing a two-week detox plan to alleviate symptoms of acid reflux, identify trigger foods to avoid, incorporate alkaline water into your daily routine, experiment with pH balancing techniques, embrace change by cultivating a positive mindset, and transition to a reflux-friendly lifestyle for long-term digestive wellness.

## Designing a Two-Week Detox Plan

A two-week detox plan offers an opportunity to reset your digestive system, reduce inflammation, and alleviate symptoms of acid reflux. By eliminating trigger foods, incorporating alkaline-rich foods and beverages, and prioritizing digestive support, you can jumpstart your journey towards optimal digestive health and well-being.

### Week 1: Elimination Phase

During the first week of the detox plan, focus on eliminating trigger foods that may exacerbate symptoms of acid reflux. Common trigger foods include spicy foods, acidic foods, caffeine, alcohol, fried foods, processed foods, and high-fat foods. By removing these potential irritants from your diet, you can reduce inflammation, alleviate symptoms, and create a foundation for digestive healing.

### Week 2: Reintroduction Phase

In the second week of the detox plan, gradually reintroduce eliminated foods one at a time and observe how your body responds. Pay attention to any changes in symptoms, such as heartburn, regurgitation, bloating, or discomfort, after reintroducing specific foods. This process helps identify trigger foods that may contribute to acid reflux and allows you to make informed dietary choices moving forward.

## Identifying Trigger Foods to Avoid

Identifying trigger foods that exacerbate symptoms of acid reflux is essential for managing the condition and promoting digestive wellness. Common trigger foods vary from person to person but may include:

- Spicy foods: Spices such as chili peppers, hot sauce, and curry can irritate the esophagus and exacerbate symptoms of acid reflux.
- Acidic foods: Citrus fruits, tomatoes, vinegar, and citrus juices can increase acidity in the stomach and trigger reflux symptoms.
- Caffeine: Coffee, tea, chocolate, and energy drinks contain caffeine, which relaxes the lower esophageal sphincter and promotes acid reflux.

- Alcohol: Alcoholic beverages, particularly wine, beer, and spirits, can relax the esophageal sphincter and increase stomach acid production, leading to reflux symptoms.
- Fried and fatty foods: Fried foods, high-fat meats, and greasy snacks are difficult to digest and may delay stomach emptying, increasing the risk of acid reflux.

By identifying and avoiding trigger foods that contribute to acid reflux, you can minimize symptom severity, reduce inflammation, and support digestive comfort.

## Incorporating Alkaline Water into Daily Routine

Incorporating alkaline water into your daily routine can help neutralize excess stomach acid, reduce acidity in the body, and alleviate symptoms of acid reflux. Alkaline water has a higher pH level than regular tap water and may offer potential benefits for digestive health and hydration. Alkaline water is believed to help neutralize acid in the stomach, creating a more alkaline environment that may reduce the risk of acid reflux and promote digestive comfort. Additionally, alkaline water is thought to provide antioxidant properties, support hydration, and contribute to overall well-being.

To incorporate alkaline water into your daily routine, consider investing in a water ionizer or alkaline water filter system that can adjust the pH level of your drinking water. Aim to consume alkaline water between meals and throughout the day to stay hydrated and support digestive wellness.

## Experimenting with pH Balancing Techniques

pH balancing techniques can help regulate acidity levels in the body, promote alkalinity, and support digestive health. By incorporating alkaline-rich foods and beverages into your diet, practicing mindful eating habits, and prioritizing stress management techniques, you can optimize pH balance and reduce the risk of acid reflux.

**Alkaline-Rich Foods**: Incorporate alkaline-rich foods such as leafy greens, cruciferous vegetables, fruits, nuts, seeds, and legumes into your diet to promote alkalinity and reduce acidity in the body.

**Mindful Eating**: Practice mindful eating habits such as chewing slowly, savoring each bite, and paying attention to hunger and fullness cues to support optimal digestion and pH balance.

**Stress Management**: Prioritize stress management techniques such as deep breathing, meditation, yoga, and relaxation exercises to reduce stress levels, promote alkalinity, and support digestive wellness.

By experimenting with pH balancing techniques and incorporating alkaline-rich foods and beverages into your daily routine, you can create a more alkaline environment in the body, reduce acidity, and support digestive comfort.

## **Embracing Change: Cultivating a Positive Mindset**

Embracing change and cultivating a positive mindset are essential components of a successful acid reflux detox journey. By reframing challenges as opportunities for growth, practicing self-compassion, and focusing on progress rather than perfection, you can navigate the complexities of digestive health with resilience and optimism.

**Mindfulness**: Practice mindfulness techniques such as meditation, gratitude journaling, and positive affirmations to cultivate a sense of presence, awareness, and acceptance in the present moment.

**Self-Compassion**: Be kind and compassionate towards yourself, especially during times of difficulty or setbacks. Acknowledge your efforts, celebrate small victories, and treat yourself with the same kindness and understanding you would offer to a loved one.

**Optimism**: Maintain a positive outlook and belief in your ability to overcome challenges and achieve your health goals. Surround yourself with supportive individuals, seek inspiration from success stories, and stay focused on the possibilities for growth and transformation.

By embracing change, cultivating a positive mindset, and practicing self-care, you can navigate the acid reflux detox journey with confidence, resilience, and grace.

## **Transitioning to a Reflux-Friendly Lifestyle**

Transitioning to a reflux-friendly lifestyle involves making sustainable changes to your diet, habits, and environment to support digestive wellness and minimize symptoms of acid reflux. By prioritizing nutrient-dense foods, practicing mindful eating, managing stress, and incorporating self-care practices into your daily routine, you can create a lifestyle that promotes optimal digestive health and well-being.

**Dietary Modifications**: Make gradual changes to your diet by incorporating reflux-friendly foods such as lean proteins, fruits, vegetables, whole grains, and alkaline-rich beverages. Minimize or avoid trigger foods that exacerbate symptoms of acid reflux, and prioritize portion control and mindful eating habits.

**Stress Management**: Implement stress management techniques such as deep breathing, meditation, yoga, and relaxation exercises to reduce stress levels, promote relaxation, and support digestive comfort.

**Physical Activity**: Engage in regular physical activity such as walking, swimming, cycling, or yoga to promote circulation, improve digestion, and support overall well-being.

**Sleep Hygiene**: Prioritize good sleep hygiene practices such as maintaining a consistent sleep schedule, creating a relaxing bedtime routine, and optimizing sleep environment to promote restful and rejuvenating sleep.

By transitioning to a reflux-friendly lifestyle, you can create an environment that supports optimal digestive health, reduces symptoms of acid reflux, and enhances overall well-being.

In conclusion, designing a two-week detox plan, identifying trigger foods to avoid, incorporating alkaline water into your daily routine, experimenting with pH balancing techniques, embracing change by cultivating a positive mindset, and transitioning to a reflux-friendly lifestyle are essential components of effective acid reflux management and digestive wellness.

By implementing targeted strategies, making informed dietary choices, and prioritizing self-care practices, you can reclaim control over your digestive health, alleviate symptoms of acid reflux, and embrace a lifestyle of balance, vitality, and well-being. In the chapters ahead, we will delve deeper into practical strategies, empowering insights, and delicious recipes to help you thrive on your journey towards optimal digestive health and vitality.
Together, let us navigate the path towards digestive wellness and embrace the transformative power of self-care, knowledge, and empowerment in reclaiming our health and vitality.

# Chapter 6: Navigating the Transition Period with Ease

Welcome to Chapter 6 of our journey towards understanding acid reflux and embracing digestive health. In this chapter, we will explore strategies for navigating the transition period with ease, practical tips for dining out and social situations, building support systems and seeking community, overcoming challenges with confidence and resilience, celebrating progress, and sustaining wellness in the maintenance phase of your acid reflux journey.

## Navigating the Transition Period with Ease

The transition period marks a significant phase in your acid reflux journey, characterized by adjustments to dietary habits, lifestyle choices, and social interactions. As you implement changes to support digestive wellness and alleviate symptoms of acid reflux, it is important to approach the transition period with patience, flexibility, and self-compassion.

**Gradual Implementation**: Transitioning to a reflux-friendly lifestyle involves gradual implementation of dietary modifications, lifestyle changes, and stress management techniques. Rather than making drastic changes overnight, focus on incorporating small, sustainable adjustments into your daily routine.

**Mindful Awareness**: Cultivate mindful awareness of your body's signals, symptoms, and reactions to different foods, environments, and stressors. Pay attention to how your body responds to dietary choices, physical activity, and stress levels, and adjust your approach accordingly.

**Self-Compassion**: Practice self-compassion and kindness towards yourself during the transition period. Embrace the process of trial and error, celebrate small victories, and acknowledge the progress you have made towards improving your digestive health and well-being.

## Practical Tips for Dining Out and Social Situations

Dining out and social situations can present challenges for individuals managing acid reflux, but with careful planning and preparation, you can navigate these occasions with confidence and ease.

**Menu Selection**: Prior to dining out, review the menu online and identify reflux-friendly options such as grilled proteins, steamed vegetables, salads with dressing on the side, and whole grains. Choose dishes that are lower in fat, spices, and acidity to minimize the risk of triggering reflux symptoms.

**Customization**: Don't hesitate to request modifications to menu items to better suit your dietary needs and preferences. Ask for sauces, dressings, and toppings on the side, opt for steamed or grilled preparations, and inquire about ingredient substitutions or omissions to accommodate your reflux-friendly diet.

**Portion Control**: Practice portion control by sharing meals with dining companions, ordering appetizers or small plates, or requesting a half portion of entrees. Listen to your body's hunger and fullness cues, and stop eating when you feel satisfied to prevent overeating and discomfort.

**Mindful Eating**: Practice mindful eating habits such as chewing slowly, savoring each bite, and paying attention to hunger and fullness cues. Minimize distractions during meals, engage in conversation with dining companions, and focus on the sensory experience of eating to enhance satisfaction and digestion.

By implementing practical tips and strategies for dining out and social situations, you can enjoy flavorful meals, connect with others, and maintain adherence to your reflux-friendly diet.

## Building Support Systems and Seeking Community

Building support systems and seeking community can provide invaluable resources, encouragement, and understanding as you navigate the challenges of managing acid reflux.

**Family and Friends**: Share your experiences, challenges, and goals with supportive family members and friends who can offer empathy, encouragement, and practical assistance. Invite loved ones to join you in exploring reflux-friendly recipes, dining out at reflux-friendly restaurants, and participating in stress-relieving activities together.

**Online Communities**: Join online support groups, forums, and social media communities dedicated to acid reflux management and digestive wellness. Connect with individuals who share similar experiences, exchange advice, and find inspiration from success stories and shared journeys.

**Healthcare Providers**: Seek guidance and support from healthcare providers, including gastroenterologists, registered dietitians, and therapists, who specialize in acid reflux management and digestive health. Discuss your concerns, treatment options, and goals for managing acid reflux, and collaborate with healthcare professionals to develop a personalized plan of care.

**Support Groups**: Consider participating in local or virtual support groups for individuals with acid reflux or related digestive disorders. Attend meetings, workshops, or educational events to learn from experts, share strategies for coping with reflux symptoms, and foster a sense of camaraderie and belonging within the reflux community.

By building support systems and seeking community, you can gain valuable insights, encouragement, and validation as you navigate the complexities of managing acid reflux and embracing digestive wellness.

# Overcoming Challenges with Confidence and Resilience

Overcoming challenges with confidence and resilience is an essential skill for navigating the ups and downs of managing acid reflux and maintaining a reflux-friendly lifestyle.

**Positive Mindset**: Cultivate a positive mindset and belief in your ability to overcome obstacles and achieve your health goals. Focus on the progress you have made, rather than dwelling on setbacks or perceived failures, and approach challenges with curiosity, creativity, and determination.

**Problem-Solving Skills**: Develop problem-solving skills to address challenges and barriers to adherence to your reflux-friendly diet and lifestyle. Brainstorm alternative solutions, seek advice from trusted sources, and remain open to trying new approaches to achieve optimal digestive health and well-being.

**Flexibility**: Embrace flexibility and adaptability in your approach to managing acid reflux. Recognize that dietary needs, lifestyle preferences, and symptom severity may vary over time, and be willing to adjust your strategies and goals accordingly to meet your evolving needs.

**Resilience**: Cultivate resilience by practicing self-care, coping strategies, and stress management techniques that promote emotional well-being and inner strength. Build a toolkit of resilience-building practices such as mindfulness, gratitude, self-compassion, and social support to navigate challenges with grace and fortitude.

By overcoming challenges with confidence and resilience, you can navigate the complexities of managing acid reflux with grace, determination, and optimism.

# Celebrating Progress: Small Victories Matter

Celebrating progress, no matter how small, is an important aspect of maintaining motivation, confidence, and momentum on your acid reflux journey.

**Acknowledge Achievements**: Take time to acknowledge and celebrate your achievements, milestones, and successes in managing acid reflux and embracing a reflux-friendly lifestyle. Recognize the efforts you have made, the changes you have implemented, and the improvements you have experienced in your digestive health and well-being.

**Set Realistic Goals**: Set realistic, achievable goals for yourself that reflect your values, priorities, and aspirations for managing acid reflux. Break larger goals into smaller, actionable steps, and celebrate each milestone along the way to maintain motivation and momentum.

**Express Gratitude**: Practice gratitude and appreciation for the progress you have made and the support you have received from others on your acid reflux journey. Express gratitude through journaling, verbal affirmations, or acts of kindness to cultivate a sense of abundance, fulfillment, and positivity in your life.

**Share Successes**: Share your successes, challenges, and insights with supportive family members, friends, or online communities who can offer encouragement, validation, and celebration of your achievements. Celebrate together as a community, and inspire others to embrace their own journeys towards digestive wellness.

By celebrating progress and embracing the journey towards optimal digestive health, you can cultivate a sense of accomplishment, empowerment, and fulfillment in managing acid reflux and reclaiming your vitality.

## Sustaining Wellness: The Maintenance Phase

Sustaining wellness in the maintenance phase involves integrating reflux-friendly habits, routines, and practices into your daily life to promote long-term digestive health and well-being.

**Consistency**: Prioritize consistency in your reflux-friendly habits, dietary choices, and lifestyle practices to maintain stability and support digestive wellness over time. Establish daily routines, meal plans, and self-care rituals that align with your goals and values for managing acid reflux.

**Self-Monitoring**: Monitor your symptoms, dietary intake, stress levels, and lifestyle habits regularly to track changes, identify triggers, and maintain awareness of your digestive health. Keep a food diary, symptom journal, or wellness tracker to record your experiences and insights on managing acid reflux.

**Adaptability**: Remain adaptable and open to adjustments in your reflux-friendly diet and lifestyle as your needs, preferences, and circumstances evolve over time. Be willing to experiment with new foods, recipes, and strategies for managing symptoms, and seek guidance from healthcare professionals as needed to optimize your approach.

**Lifelong Learning**: Embrace a mindset of lifelong learning and growth in your journey towards optimal digestive health and well-being. Stay informed about advances in acid reflux research, treatment options, and holistic approaches to digestive wellness, and seek opportunities for education, exploration, and self-discovery.

By sustaining wellness in the maintenance phase, you can cultivate resilience, vitality, and balance in managing acid reflux and living a life of optimal digestive health and well-being.

In conclusion, navigating the transition period with ease, implementing practical tips for dining out and social situations, building support systems and seeking community, overcoming challenges with confidence and resilience, celebrating progress, and sustaining wellness in the maintenance phase are essential components of managing acid reflux and embracing digestive health.

By embracing a holistic approach to acid reflux management, prioritizing self-care practices, and fostering connections within the reflux community, you can navigate the complexities of digestive health with grace, resilience, and vitality. In the chapters ahead, we will delve deeper into practical strategies, empowering insights, and delicious recipes to help you thrive on your journey towards optimal digestive health and vitality.

Together, let us navigate the path towards digestive wellness and embrace the transformative power of self-care, knowledge, and empowerment in reclaiming our health and vitality.

# Chapter 7: Crafting Delicious and Nutritious Meal Plans

Welcome to Chapter 7 of our journey towards understanding acid reflux and embracing digestive health. In this chapter, we will explore the art of crafting delicious and nutritious meal plans that support optimal digestive health, embracing variety and creativity in cooking, stocking up on reflux-friendly pantry staples, incorporating physical activity into your daily routine, cultivating a healthy relationship with food, and unlocking the secrets of longevity through mindful nutrition and lifestyle choices.

## Crafting Delicious and Nutritious Meal Plans

Crafting delicious and nutritious meal plans is essential for managing acid reflux and promoting digestive wellness. By prioritizing whole, nutrient-dense foods and minimizing triggers that exacerbate reflux symptoms, you can create meals that nourish your body, support optimal digestion, and enhance overall well-being.

**Balanced Macronutrients**: Design meal plans that include a balance of macronutrients, including carbohydrates, proteins, and healthy fats, to provide sustained energy, promote satiety, and support metabolic health. Incorporate a variety of colorful fruits and vegetables, lean proteins such as poultry, fish, and legumes, and healthy fats from sources like nuts, seeds, and avocado.

**Fiber-Rich Foods**: Include plenty of fiber-rich foods such as whole grains, legumes, fruits, and vegetables in your meal plans to support digestive health, regulate bowel movements, and promote feelings of fullness and satisfaction. Aim for a diverse range of fiber sources to ensure adequate intake of soluble and insoluble fiber.

**Hydration**: Stay hydrated throughout the day by incorporating water, herbal teas, and hydrating foods such as fruits and vegetables into your meal plans. Adequate hydration supports digestion, nutrient absorption, and overall well-being, and can help alleviate symptoms of acid reflux by promoting optimal stomach function.

**Mindful Eating**: Practice mindful eating habits such as chewing slowly, savoring each bite, and paying attention to hunger and fullness cues to enhance digestion, prevent overeating, and promote satisfaction with meals. Create a calm, distraction-free environment for eating, and focus on the sensory experience of food to foster a deeper connection with your meals.

By crafting delicious and nutritious meal plans that prioritize whole, nourishing foods and mindful eating practices, you can support digestive wellness, alleviate symptoms of acid reflux, and enjoy a varied and satisfying diet.

## Embracing Variety and Creativity in Cooking

Embracing variety and creativity in cooking is key to maintaining enjoyment and satisfaction with your reflux-friendly diet. Experimenting with new ingredients, flavors, and cooking techniques can help keep meals interesting and flavorful, while also providing a wealth of nutrients and health benefits.

**Explore Global Cuisines**: Explore the diverse world of global cuisines and incorporate flavors and ingredients from different cultures into your cooking repertoire. Experiment with Mediterranean, Asian, Latin American, and Middle Eastern cuisines, which often feature plant-based ingredients, fresh herbs, and aromatic spices that add depth and complexity to dishes.

**Plant-Based Proteins**: Experiment with plant-based protein sources such as tofu, tempeh, lentils, chickpeas, and beans to add variety and nutrient diversity to your meals. Plant-based proteins are rich in fiber, vitamins, minerals, and phytonutrients, and can be incorporated into a wide range of dishes, from salads and stir-fries to soups and stews.

**Herbs and Spices**: Enhance the flavor and nutritional profile of your meals by incorporating a variety of herbs, spices, and aromatic seasonings. Experiment with fresh herbs such as basil, cilantro, mint, and parsley, as well as spices like turmeric, ginger, cumin, and cinnamon, to add depth, complexity, and antioxidant-rich flavor to your dishes.

**Creative Cooking Techniques**: Get creative in the kitchen by exploring new cooking techniques such as grilling, roasting, steaming, sautéing, and braising to enhance the natural flavors and textures of ingredients. Experiment with different methods of food preparation to discover your favorite cooking styles and techniques.
By embracing variety and creativity in cooking, you can transform mealtime into a joyful and fulfilling experience, while also nourishing your body with nutrient-rich foods and flavorful dishes.

## Stocking Up on Reflux-Friendly Pantry Staples

Stocking up on reflux-friendly pantry staples is essential for maintaining a well-stocked kitchen and preparing delicious and nutritious meals that support digestive health and alleviate symptoms of acid reflux.

**Whole Grains**: Keep a variety of whole grains such as brown rice, quinoa, oats, barley, and whole wheat pasta on hand to use as the foundation for nutritious and filling meals. Whole grains are rich in fiber, vitamins, minerals, and antioxidants, and can help promote digestive health and regulate blood sugar levels.

**Canned and Dried Beans**: Stock your pantry with canned and dried beans such as chickpeas, black beans, kidney beans, and lentils, which are versatile, affordable, and nutrient-dense sources of plant-based protein, fiber, and essential nutrients. Rinse canned beans before using to reduce sodium content and improve digestibility.

**Healthy Oils**: Choose healthy oils such as olive oil, avocado oil, coconut oil, and sesame oil for cooking, baking, and dressing salads. Healthy oils provide heart-healthy fats, antioxidants, and anti-inflammatory compounds that support overall health and well-being.

**Canned Tomatoes and Tomato Products**: Opt for canned tomatoes and tomato products such as tomato sauce, diced tomatoes, and tomato paste that are free from added sugars and preservatives. Tomatoes are a rich source of vitamins, minerals, and antioxidants, but can be acidic and trigger reflux symptoms in some individuals, so moderation is key.

**Low-Acidic Foods**: Include low-acidic foods such as canned fruits in water or natural juice, unsweetened applesauce, and low-acidic vegetables such as carrots, cucumbers, and bell peppers in your pantry for convenient and nutritious snacking options.
By stocking up on reflux-friendly pantry staples, you can streamline meal preparation, minimize the need for last-minute trips to the grocery store, and ensure that you always have nutritious ingredients on hand to create satisfying and wholesome meals.

## Incorporating Physical Activity into Daily Routine

Incorporating physical activity into your daily routine is essential for promoting overall health and well-being, supporting digestive function, and managing symptoms of acid reflux. Regular exercise can help improve digestion, reduce stress levels, support weight management, and enhance mood and energy levels.

**Aerobic Exercise**: Engage in aerobic activities such as walking, jogging, swimming, cycling, or dancing for at least 30 minutes most days of the week to promote cardiovascular health, boost metabolism, and support digestive function. Choose activities that you enjoy and that fit your fitness level and preferences.

**Strength Training**: Incorporate strength training exercises such as weightlifting, resistance band exercises, or bodyweight exercises into your fitness routine to build muscle mass, increase metabolism, and improve overall strength and endurance. Aim to include strength training exercises at least two days per week, targeting major muscle groups.

**Flexibility and Balance**: Include flexibility and balance exercises such as yoga, Pilates, tai chi, or stretching routines to improve range of motion, enhance posture, and reduce muscle tension and stiffness. Incorporate gentle stretching and relaxation techniques into your daily routine to promote relaxation, stress reduction, and overall well-being.

**Outdoor Activities**: Take advantage of outdoor activities such as hiking, gardening, or playing sports with friends and family to enjoy the benefits of fresh air, sunshine, and nature. Outdoor activities can invigorate the mind, reduce stress, and promote feelings of vitality and connection with the natural world.
By incorporating physical activity into your daily routine, you can enhance digestive health, promote overall well-being, and reduce the risk of reflux symptoms and complications.

# Cultivating a Healthy Relationship with Food

Cultivating a healthy relationship with food is essential for nourishing your body, mind, and spirit, and fostering a positive and sustainable approach to eating that supports digestive health and overall well-being.

**Mindful Eating**: Practice mindful eating habits such as paying attention to hunger and fullness cues, savoring each bite, and cultivating awareness of the sensory experience of food. Avoid distractions such as screens, multitasking, or eating on the go, and instead focus on the pleasure and nourishment that food provides.

**Intuitive Eating**: Embrace intuitive eating principles by listening to your body's signals, cravings, and preferences, and honoring your hunger and fullness cues without judgment or restriction. Trust your body to guide you towards foods that satisfy your nutritional needs and support your overall health and well-being.

**Food as Fuel**: View food as fuel for your body and mind, providing essential nutrients, energy, and nourishment for optimal function and vitality. Choose foods that make you feel energized, satisfied, and nourished, and prioritize nutrient-dense, whole foods that support digestive health and overall well-being.

**Emotional Eating**: Recognize the role of emotions, stress, and environmental cues in influencing eating behaviors, and develop healthy coping strategies and alternatives to emotional eating. Practice self-care activities such as journaling, meditation, deep breathing, or engaging in hobbies and interests to manage stress and emotions without turning to food.

By cultivating a healthy relationship with food based on mindfulness, intuition, and self-care, you can foster a positive and sustainable approach to eating that supports digestive health, enhances overall well-being, and nurtures a sense of joy and fulfillment in nourishing your body and soul.

# Unlocking the Secrets of Longevity

Unlocking the secrets of longevity involves embracing holistic lifestyle practices, dietary habits, and mindset shifts that promote optimal health, vitality, and well-being throughout the lifespan. By prioritizing self-care, stress management, social connections, and purposeful living, you can enhance longevity and quality of life.

**Nutrient-Rich Diet**: Adopt a nutrient-rich diet that prioritizes whole, minimally processed foods such as fruits, vegetables, whole grains, lean proteins, and healthy fats. Choose foods that are rich in vitamins, minerals, antioxidants, and phytonutrients to support immune function, reduce inflammation, and promote cellular health and longevity.

**Anti-Inflammatory Foods**: Incorporate anti-inflammatory foods such as fatty fish, nuts, seeds, olive oil, berries, leafy greens, and turmeric into your diet to reduce inflammation, support heart health, and enhance longevity. Minimize intake of processed foods, sugary snacks, refined carbohydrates, and trans fats that can promote inflammation and accelerate aging.

**Physical Activity**: Engage in regular physical activity and exercise to promote cardiovascular health, maintain muscle mass and strength, and support cognitive function and mental well-being. Aim for a combination of aerobic exercise, strength training, flexibility, and balance exercises to enhance overall fitness and longevity.

**Stress Management**: Prioritize stress management techniques such as mindfulness meditation, deep breathing exercises, yoga, tai chi, or nature walks to reduce stress levels, promote relaxation, and support emotional resilience and well-being. Cultivate a sense of calm, balance, and inner peace amidst life's challenges and transitions.

**Social Connections**: Nurture meaningful social connections and relationships with family, friends, and community members to foster a sense of belonging, connection, and purpose in life. Prioritize quality time spent with loved ones, engage in meaningful conversations and shared activities, and seek out opportunities for connection and camaraderie.

**Purposeful Living**: Discover and cultivate a sense of purpose, meaning, and fulfillment in your life by pursuing activities, interests, and goals that align with your values, passions, and strengths. Engage in volunteer work, creative endeavors, or lifelong learning opportunities that bring joy, fulfillment, and a sense of contribution to your life and the lives of others.
By unlocking the secrets of longevity through holistic lifestyle practices, dietary habits, and mindset shifts, you can cultivate a life of vitality, purpose, and well-being that extends far beyond the number of years lived.

In conclusion, crafting delicious and nutritious meal plans, embracing variety and creativity in cooking, stocking up on reflux-friendly pantry staples, incorporating physical activity into your daily routine, cultivating a healthy relationship with food, and unlocking the secrets of longevity are essential components of managing acid reflux, promoting digestive health, and enhancing overall well-being.

By embracing mindful nutrition and lifestyle practices, you can nourish your body, mind, and spirit, and embark on a journey towards optimal health, vitality, and longevity. In the chapters ahead, we will delve deeper into practical strategies, empowering insights, and delicious recipes to help you thrive on your journey towards digestive health and vitality.
Together, let us unlock the secrets of longevity and embrace the transformative power of holistic wellness in reclaiming our health, vitality, and well-being.

# Healthy Breakfast Recipes

## Banana Oatmeal Pancakes

*Introduction:* These fluffy pancakes combine the natural sweetness of bananas with hearty oats for a nutritious breakfast option.
*Prep Time:* 20 minutes

*Ingredients:*
- 1 ripe banana
- 1 cup rolled oats
- 1 egg
- 1/2 teaspoon cinnamon
- 1/2 teaspoon vanilla extract
- 1/4 cup milk (any type)
- 1 teaspoon baking powder
- Pinch of salt

*Instructions:*
1. Mash the banana in a bowl until smooth.
2. Add oats, egg, cinnamon, vanilla extract, milk, baking powder, and salt. Mix until well combined.
3. Heat a non-stick skillet over medium heat and lightly grease with oil or cooking spray.
4. Pour 1/4 cup of batter onto the skillet for each pancake.
5. Cook until bubbles form on the surface, then flip and cook until golden brown on both sides.
6. Serve warm with your favorite toppings.

*Nutritional Information:* (per serving)
- Calories: 180
- Protein: 7g
- Carbohydrates: 30g
- Fat: 4g
- Fiber: 4g

## Greek Yogurt Parfait with Berries and Honey

*Introduction:* This parfait is a delightful combination of creamy Greek yogurt, fresh berries, and a drizzle of honey, perfect for a quick and nutritious breakfast.
*Prep Time:* 10 minutes

*Ingredients:*
- 1 cup Greek yogurt
- 1/2 cup mixed berries (such as strawberries, blueberries, raspberries)

- 1 tablespoon honey
- Granola (optional)

*Instructions:*
1. In a glass or bowl, layer Greek yogurt, mixed berries, and drizzle with honey.
2. Repeat the layers until ingredients are used up.
3. Top with granola for added crunch if desired.
4. Serve immediately and enjoy!

*Nutritional Information:* (per serving)
- Calories: 220
- Protein: 18g
- Carbohydrates: 35g
- Fat: 3g
- Fiber: 4g

## **Quinoa Breakfast Bowl with Almond Milk and Fruit**

*Introduction:* This nutritious breakfast bowl features protein-packed quinoa, creamy almond milk, and a medley of fresh fruits for a satisfying start to your day.
*Prep Time:* 15 minutes

*Ingredients:*
- 1/2 cup cooked quinoa
- 1/2 cup almond milk
- 1/2 cup mixed fruit (such as sliced banana, berries, diced mango)
- 1 tablespoon honey or maple syrup (optional)
- Chopped nuts or seeds (optional)

*Instructions:*
1. In a bowl, combine cooked quinoa and almond milk.
2. Top with mixed fruit and drizzle with honey or maple syrup if desired.
3. Sprinkle with chopped nuts or seeds for extra crunch.
4. Serve immediately and enjoy this wholesome breakfast bowl.

*Nutritional Information:* (per serving)
- Calories: 250
- Protein: 8g
- Carbohydrates: 45g
- Fat: 5g
- Fiber: 6g

## Whole Grain Toast with Almond Butter and Sliced Banana

*Introduction:* Simple yet satisfying, this toast is a nutritious combination of whole grain bread, creamy almond butter, and fresh banana slices.
*Prep Time:* 5 minutes

*Ingredients:*
- 2 slices whole grain bread, toasted
- 2 tablespoons almond butter
- 1 ripe banana, sliced
- Honey (optional)
- Chia seeds (optional)

*Instructions:*
1. Spread almond butter evenly on each slice of toasted whole grain bread.
2. Arrange banana slices on top of the almond butter.
3. Drizzle with honey and sprinkle with chia seeds if desired.
4. Serve immediately for a quick and wholesome breakfast.

*Nutritional Information:* (per serving)
- Calories: 320
- Protein: 9g
- Carbohydrates: 45g
- Fat: 14g
- Fiber: 8g

## Muesli with Yogurt and Sliced Peaches

*Introduction:* This muesli breakfast combines crunchy oats, creamy yogurt, and juicy peaches for a refreshing and nutritious morning meal.
*Prep Time:* 10 minutes

*Ingredients:*
- 1/2 cup muesli or rolled oats
- 1/2 cup plain yogurt
- 1 ripe peach, sliced
- Honey or maple syrup (optional)
- Almonds or walnuts, chopped (optional)

*Instructions:*
1. In a bowl, combine muesli or rolled oats with plain yogurt.
2. Top with sliced peaches.
3. Drizzle with honey or maple syrup if desired.
4. Garnish with chopped almonds or walnuts for added texture.

5. Serve immediately and enjoy this wholesome breakfast.

*Nutritional Information:* (per serving)
- Calories: 280
- Protein: 9g
- Carbohydrates: 45g
- Fat: 7g
- Fiber: 6g

## Avocado Toast with Tomato and Sprouts

*Introduction:* This avocado toast is a delicious and nutritious way to start your day, featuring creamy avocado, ripe tomatoes, and crunchy sprouts.
*Prep Time:* 10 minutes

*Ingredients:*
- 2 slices whole grain bread, toasted
- 1 ripe avocado, mashed
- 1 ripe tomato, sliced
- Sprouts (such as alfalfa or broccoli)
- Lemon juice
- Salt and pepper to taste

*Instructions:*
1. Spread mashed avocado evenly on each slice of toasted whole grain bread.
2. Top with sliced tomatoes and sprouts.
3. Squeeze fresh lemon juice over the toppings.
4. Season with salt and pepper to taste.
5. Serve immediately for a delicious and nutritious breakfast.

*Nutritional Information:* (per serving)
- Calories: 280
- Protein: 8g
- Carbohydrates: 35g
- Fat: 14g
- Fiber: 10g

## Apple Cinnamon Overnight Oats

*Introduction:* These overnight oats are a convenient and flavorful breakfast option, combining the sweetness of apples with warm cinnamon spice.
*Prep Time:* 5 minutes (plus overnight chilling)

*Ingredients:*
- 1/2 cup rolled oats
- 1/2 cup almond milk
- 1/2 apple, diced
- 1 tablespoon maple syrup or honey
- 1/2 teaspoon cinnamon
- Chopped nuts or seeds (optional)

*Instructions:*
1. In a jar or bowl, combine rolled oats, almond milk, diced apple, maple syrup or honey, and cinnamon.
2. Stir well to combine all ingredients.
3. Cover and refrigerate overnight.
4. In the morning, give the oats a good stir.
5. Top with chopped nuts or seeds if desired.
6. Serve chilled and enjoy!

*Nutritional Information:* (per serving)
- Calories: 280
- Protein: 7g
- Carbohydrates: 50g
- Fat: 6g
- Fiber: 8g

## Veggie Omelette with Goat Cheese

*Introduction:* This veggie omelette is loaded with colorful vegetables and creamy goat cheese, making it a satisfying and nutritious breakfast choice.
*Prep Time:* 15 minutes

*Ingredients:*
- 2 eggs
- 1/4 cup bell peppers, diced
- 1/4 cup spinach, chopped
- 2 tablespoons red onion, finely chopped
- 2 tablespoons goat cheese, crumbled
- Salt and pepper to taste
- Olive oil or butter for cooking

*Instructions:*
1. In a bowl, whisk together eggs, bell peppers, spinach, red onion, salt, and pepper.
2. Heat olive oil or butter in a non-stick skillet over medium heat.
3. Pour the egg mixture into the skillet and cook until the edges start to set.
4. Sprinkle crumbled goat cheese over one half of the omelette.

5.  Carefully fold the omelette in half and cook for another minute until the cheese melts.
6.  Slide the omelette onto a plate and serve hot.

*Nutritional Information:* (per serving)
- Calories: 220
- Protein: 14g
- Carbohydrates: 5g
- Fat: 15g
- Fiber: 2g

## Buckwheat Porridge with Sliced Strawberries

*Introduction:* This buckwheat porridge is a hearty and nutritious breakfast option, topped with sweet sliced strawberries for a burst of flavor.
*Prep Time:* 20 minutes

*Ingredients:*
- 1/2 cup buckwheat groats
- 1 1/2 cups water or milk (any type)
- Pinch of salt
- 1/2 cup sliced strawberries
- Honey or maple syrup (optional)
- Chopped nuts or seeds (optional)

*Instructions:*
1.  Rinse the buckwheat groats under cold water.
2.  In a saucepan, bring water or milk to a boil.
3.  Add buckwheat groats and a pinch of salt to the boiling liquid.
4.  Reduce heat to low, cover, and simmer for 15-20 minutes, or until the groats are tender.
5.  Remove from heat and let it sit for a few minutes.
6.  Serve the porridge hot, topped with sliced strawberries.
7.  Drizzle with honey or maple syrup and sprinkle with chopped nuts or seeds if desired.

*Nutritional Information:* (per serving)
- Calories: 250
- Protein: 8g
- Carbohydrates: 45g
- Fat: 3g
- Fiber: 6g

## Smoothie Bowl with Mixed Berries and Granola

*Introduction:* This smoothie bowl is packed with antioxidants and nutrients from mixed berries, topped with crunchy granola for a satisfying breakfast.

*Prep Time:* 10 minutes

*Ingredients:*
- 1 cup mixed berries (such as strawberries, blueberries, raspberries)
- 1/2 banana, sliced
- 1/2 cup spinach or kale leaves
- 1/2 cup almond milk
- 1 tablespoon honey or maple syrup (optional)
- Granola for topping
- Chia seeds or flaxseeds (optional)

*Instructions:*
1. In a blender, combine mixed berries, banana, spinach or kale leaves, almond milk, and honey or maple syrup.
2. Blend until smooth and creamy.
3. Pour the smoothie into a bowl.
4. Top with granola and sprinkle with chia seeds or flaxseeds if desired.
5. Serve immediately and enjoy this refreshing breakfast.

*Nutritional Information:* (per serving)
- Calories: 280
- Protein: 8g
- Carbohydrates: 50g
- Fat: 6g
- Fiber: 10g

## **Peanut Butter Banana Smoothie with Flaxseed**

*Introduction:* This creamy peanut butter banana smoothie is a protein-packed breakfast option, enhanced with the nutritional benefits of flaxseed.
*Prep Time:* 5 minutes

*Ingredients:*
- 1 ripe banana
- 2 tablespoons peanut butter
- 1 cup milk (any type)
- 1 tablespoon flaxseed meal
- Honey or maple syrup (optional)
- Ice cubes (optional)

*Instructions:*
1. In a blender, combine ripe banana, peanut butter, milk, and flaxseed meal.
2. Add honey or maple syrup for sweetness if desired.
3. Add ice cubes for a colder smoothie.

4. Blend until smooth and creamy.
5. Pour into a glass and serve immediately.

*Nutritional Information:* (per serving)
- Calories: 350
- Protein: 12g
- Carbohydrates: 30g
- Fat: 20g
- Fiber: 6g

## Chia Seed Pudding with Mango and Coconut

*Introduction:* This chia seed pudding is a delightful combination of creamy coconut milk, sweet mango, and nutritious chia seeds, perfect for a healthy breakfast or snack.
*Prep Time:* 5 minutes (plus chilling time)

*Ingredients:*
- 1/4 cup chia seeds
- 1 cup coconut milk
- 1 ripe mango, diced
- Shredded coconut for garnish
- Maple syrup or honey (optional)

*Instructions:*
1. In a bowl, mix chia seeds and coconut milk.
2. Add maple syrup or honey for sweetness if desired.
3. Stir well to combine and let it sit for 5 minutes.
4. Stir the mixture again to prevent clumping.
5. Cover and refrigerate for at least 2 hours or overnight.
6. Before serving, stir the pudding and top with diced mango and shredded coconut.
7. Enjoy this creamy and nutritious chia seed pudding.

*Nutritional Information:* (per serving)
- Calories: 280
- Protein: 6g
- Carbohydrates: 30g
- Fat: 15g
- Fiber: 10g

## Almond Flour Waffles with Fresh Berries

*Introduction:* These almond flour waffles are gluten-free and deliciously crispy, topped with a medley of fresh berries for a delightful breakfast treat.
*Prep Time:* 15 minutes

*Ingredients:*
- 1 cup almond flour
- 2 eggs
- 1/4 cup milk (any type)
- 1 tablespoon maple syrup or honey
- 1/2 teaspoon baking powder
- Pinch of salt
- Fresh berries for topping
- Greek yogurt (optional)

*Instructions:*
1. Preheat waffle iron according to manufacturer's instructions.
2. In a bowl, whisk together almond flour, eggs, milk, maple syrup or honey, baking powder, and salt until smooth.
3. Pour the batter onto the preheated waffle iron and cook until golden brown and crispy.
4. Serve the waffles hot, topped with fresh berries and a dollop of Greek yogurt if desired.
5. Enjoy these gluten-free almond flour waffles for a wholesome breakfast.

*Nutritional Information:* (per serving)
- Calories: 280
- Protein: 12g
- Carbohydrates: 20g
- Fat: 18g
- Fiber: 6g

## Green Smoothie with Kale, Pineapple, and Ginger

*Introduction:* This green smoothie is packed with vitamins and antioxidants from kale, pineapple, and ginger, making it a refreshing and nutritious breakfast option.
*Prep Time:* 5 minutes

*Ingredients:*
- 1 cup kale leaves, stems removed
- 1 cup fresh or frozen pineapple chunks
- 1/2 inch fresh ginger, peeled
- 1/2 banana
- 1/2 cup coconut water or water
- Ice cubes (optional)
- Honey or maple syrup (optional)

*Instructions:*
1. In a blender, combine kale leaves, pineapple chunks, fresh ginger, banana, and coconut water or water.
2. Add honey or maple syrup for sweetness if desired.

3. Add ice cubes for a colder smoothie.
4. Blend until smooth and creamy.
5. Pour into glasses and serve immediately.

*Nutritional Information:* (per serving)
- Calories: 150
- Protein: 3g
- Carbohydrates: 35g
- Fat: 1g
- Fiber: 6g

## Quinoa Breakfast Muffins with Spinach and Feta

*Introduction:* These quinoa breakfast muffins are packed with protein and flavor from spinach, feta cheese, and nutritious quinoa, making them a perfect grab-and-go breakfast option.
*Prep Time:* 20 minutes

*Ingredients:*
- 1 cup cooked quinoa
- 1 cup fresh spinach, chopped
- 1/2 cup crumbled feta cheese
- 4 eggs
- 1/4 cup milk (any type)
- Salt and pepper to taste
- Cooking spray or olive oil for greasing muffin tin

*Instructions:*
1. Preheat oven to 350°F (175°C) and grease a muffin tin with cooking spray or olive oil.
2. In a bowl, whisk together eggs, milk, salt, and pepper.
3. Stir in cooked quinoa, chopped spinach, and crumbled feta cheese until well combined.
4. Divide the mixture evenly among the muffin cups.
5. Bake for 20-25 minutes, or until the muffins are set and golden brown on top.
6. Remove from the oven and let them cool slightly before serving.
7. Enjoy these delicious and nutritious quinoa breakfast muffins.

*Nutritional Information:* (per serving, 2 muffins)
- Calories: 200
- Protein: 12g
- Carbohydrates: 15g
- Fat: 10g
- Fiber: 2g

# Delicious Lunch Recipes

## Turkey and Avocado Wrap with Lettuce and Tomato

*Introduction:* This turkey and avocado wrap is a satisfying and healthy lunch option, filled with fresh vegetables and lean protein.
*Prep Time:* 10 minutes

*Ingredients:*
- 1 large whole wheat tortilla
- 3 slices turkey breast
- 1/2 avocado, sliced
- 2 lettuce leaves
- 1 tomato, sliced
- Mustard or mayonnaise (optional)

*Instructions:*
1. Lay the tortilla flat on a clean surface.
2. Layer turkey slices, avocado slices, lettuce leaves, and tomato slices on top of the tortilla.
3. Add mustard or mayonnaise if desired.
4. Roll the tortilla tightly into a wrap.
5. Cut the wrap in half and serve immediately.

*Nutritional Information:* (per serving)
- Calories: 350
- Protein: 20g
- Carbohydrates: 30g
- Fat: 18g
- Fiber: 8g

## Quinoa Salad with Cucumber, Tomato, and Lemon Vinaigrette

*Introduction:* This quinoa salad is packed with fresh vegetables and tossed in a tangy lemon vinaigrette, making it a light and refreshing lunch option.
*Prep Time:* 20 minutes

*Ingredients:*
- 1 cup cooked quinoa
- 1 cucumber, diced
- 1 tomato, diced
- 1/4 cup red onion, finely chopped
- 1/4 cup fresh parsley, chopped
- 2 tablespoons lemon juice
- 2 tablespoons olive oil

- Salt and pepper to taste

*Instructions:*
1. In a large bowl, combine cooked quinoa, diced cucumber, diced tomato, chopped red onion, and chopped parsley.
2. In a small bowl, whisk together lemon juice, olive oil, salt, and pepper to make the vinaigrette.
3. Pour the vinaigrette over the quinoa salad and toss to coat evenly.
4. Serve chilled or at room temperature.

*Nutritional Information:* (per serving)
- Calories: 250
- Protein: 6g
- Carbohydrates: 30g
- Fat: 12g
- Fiber: 5g

## Chicken and Vegetable Stir-Fry with Brown Rice

*Introduction:* This chicken and vegetable stir-fry is a quick and flavorful lunch option, packed with protein and fiber from chicken and colorful vegetables.
*Prep Time:* 20 minutes

*Ingredients:*
- 1 boneless, skinless chicken breast, thinly sliced
- 1 cup mixed vegetables (such as bell peppers, broccoli, carrots)
- 2 cups cooked brown rice
- 2 tablespoons soy sauce
- 1 tablespoon sesame oil
- 1 clove garlic, minced
- 1 teaspoon ginger, grated
- Green onions for garnish (optional)

*Instructions:*
1. Heat sesame oil in a large skillet or wok over medium-high heat.
2. Add minced garlic and grated ginger, and cook until fragrant.
3. Add sliced chicken breast and cook until browned and cooked through.
4. Add mixed vegetables to the skillet and stir-fry until tender-crisp.
5. Stir in cooked brown rice and soy sauce, and toss until well combined.
6. Cook for another 2-3 minutes, stirring occasionally.
7. Garnish with chopped green onions if desired.
8. Serve hot and enjoy this delicious chicken and vegetable stir-fry.

*Nutritional Information:* (per serving)
- Calories: 380
- Protein: 25g
- Carbohydrates: 45g
- Fat: 10g
- Fiber: 6g

## **Spinach Salad with Grilled Chicken and Balsamic Dressing**

*Introduction:* This spinach salad is loaded with grilled chicken breast and drizzled with tangy balsamic dressing, making it a satisfying and nutritious lunch option.
*Prep Time:* 15 minutes

*Ingredients:*
- 2 cups fresh spinach leaves
- 1 grilled chicken breast, sliced
- 1/4 cup cherry tomatoes, halved
- 1/4 cup cucumber, sliced
- 2 tablespoons balsamic vinegar
- 1 tablespoon olive oil
- Salt and pepper to taste

*Instructions:*
1. In a large bowl, combine fresh spinach leaves, sliced grilled chicken breast, cherry tomatoes, and cucumber slices.
2. In a small bowl, whisk together balsamic vinegar, olive oil, salt, and pepper to make the dressing.
3. Drizzle the dressing over the salad and toss gently to coat.
4. Serve immediately and enjoy this flavorful spinach salad.

*Nutritional Information:* (per serving)
- Calories: 320
- Protein: 30g
- Carbohydrates: 10g
- Fat: 15g
- Fiber: 3g

## **Hummus and Veggie Sandwich on Whole Wheat Bread**

*Introduction:* This hummus and veggie sandwich is a delicious and nutritious lunch option, featuring creamy hummus and crunchy vegetables on whole wheat bread.
*Prep Time:* 10 minutes

*Ingredients:*
- 2 slices whole wheat bread
- 2 tablespoons hummus
- 1/4 cup shredded carrots
- 1/4 cup cucumber slices
- 1/4 cup bell peppers, thinly sliced
- Baby spinach leaves
- Salt and pepper to taste

*Instructions:*
1. Spread hummus evenly on one slice of whole wheat bread.
2. Layer shredded carrots, cucumber slices, bell peppers, and baby spinach leaves on top of the hummus.
3. Season with salt and pepper to taste.
4. Top with the second slice of whole wheat bread.
5. Slice the sandwich in half and serve immediately.

*Nutritional Information:* (per serving)
- Calories: 250
- Protein: 10g
- Carbohydrates: 35g
- Fat: 8g
- Fiber: 8g

## **Cauliflower Rice Bowl with Black Beans and Avocado**

*Introduction:* This cauliflower rice bowl is a low-carb and nutrient-packed lunch option, featuring black beans, avocado, and flavorful spices.
*Prep Time:* 25 minutes

*Ingredients:*
- 2 cups cauliflower rice
- 1/2 cup black beans, drained and rinsed
- 1/2 avocado, sliced
- 1/4 cup salsa
- 1/4 cup chopped cilantro
- Lime wedges for garnish
- Salt and pepper to taste

*Instructions:*
1. Heat a skillet over medium heat and add cauliflower rice.
2. Cook, stirring occasionally, until cauliflower rice is tender, about 5-7 minutes.
3. Season cauliflower rice with salt and pepper to taste.

4. Divide cauliflower rice into bowls and top with black beans, sliced avocado, salsa, and chopped cilantro.
5. Serve with lime wedges for garnish.
6. Enjoy this delicious and nutritious cauliflower rice bowl.

*Nutritional Information:* (per serving)
- Calories: 280
- Protein: 10g
- Carbohydrates: 35g
- Fat: 12g
- Fiber: 12g

## Caprese Salad with Fresh Mozzarella and Basil

*Introduction:* This Caprese salad is a classic Italian dish featuring fresh mozzarella, ripe tomatoes, and fragrant basil, drizzled with balsamic glaze.
*Prep Time:* 10 minutes

*Ingredients:*
- 1 large ripe tomato, sliced
- 4 ounces fresh mozzarella cheese, sliced
- Fresh basil leaves
- Balsamic glaze
- Extra virgin olive oil
- Salt and pepper to taste

*Instructions:*
1. Arrange tomato slices and fresh mozzarella slices on a serving platter.
2. Tuck fresh basil leaves between the tomato and mozzarella slices.
3. Drizzle balsamic glaze and extra virgin olive oil over the salad.
4. Season with salt and pepper to taste.
5. Serve immediately and enjoy this refreshing Caprese salad.

*Nutritional Information:* (per serving)
- Calories: 250
- Protein: 15g
- Carbohydrates: 5g
- Fat: 20g
- Fiber: 1g

## Greek Chickpea Salad with Feta and Olives

*Introduction:* This Greek chickpea salad is bursting with Mediterranean flavors, featuring chickpeas, feta cheese, Kalamata olives, and a tangy lemon dressing.

*Prep Time:* 15 minutes

*Ingredients:*
- 1 can chickpeas, drained and rinsed
- 1/2 cucumber, diced
- 1/2 red onion, finely chopped
- 1/4 cup Kalamata olives, pitted and halved
- 1/4 cup crumbled feta cheese
- 2 tablespoons fresh lemon juice
- 2 tablespoons extra virgin olive oil
- 1 teaspoon dried oregano
- Salt and pepper to taste

*Instructions:*
1. In a large bowl, combine chickpeas, diced cucumber, chopped red onion, halved Kalamata olives, and crumbled feta cheese.
2. In a small bowl, whisk together fresh lemon juice, extra virgin olive oil, dried oregano, salt, and pepper to make the dressing.
3. Pour the dressing over the salad and toss gently to coat.
4. Serve chilled or at room temperature.

*Nutritional Information:* (per serving)
- Calories: 280
- Protein: 10g
- Carbohydrates: 30g
- Fat: 15g
- Fiber: 8g

## Turkey Meatballs with Zucchini Noodles and Marinara Sauce

*Introduction:* These turkey meatballs are served with spiralized zucchini noodles and marinara sauce for a low-carb and satisfying lunch option.
*Prep Time:* 30 minutes

*Ingredients:*
- 1 pound ground turkey
- 1/4 cup breadcrumbs
- 1 egg
- 2 cloves garlic, minced
- 1/4 cup grated Parmesan cheese
- Salt and pepper to taste
- 2 zucchini, spiralized
- 1 cup marinara sauce
- Fresh parsley for garnish

*Instructions:*
1. Preheat oven to 375°F (190°C) and line a baking sheet with parchment paper.
2. In a large bowl, combine ground turkey, breadcrumbs, egg, minced garlic, grated Parmesan cheese, salt, and pepper.
3. Shape the mixture into meatballs and place them on the prepared baking sheet.
4. Bake meatballs in the preheated oven for 20-25 minutes, or until cooked through and golden brown.
5. While the meatballs are baking, heat marinara sauce in a skillet over medium heat.
6. Add spiralized zucchini noodles to the skillet and toss to coat in the sauce.
7. Cook until the zucchini noodles are tender, about 5-7 minutes.
8. Serve turkey meatballs over zucchini noodles, garnished with fresh parsley.

*Nutritional Information:* (per serving)
- Calories: 320
- Protein: 25g
- Carbohydrates: 15g
- Fat: 18g
- Fiber: 4g

## **Roasted Vegetable and Quinoa Bowl with Tahini Dressing**

*Introduction:* This roasted vegetable and quinoa bowl is a hearty and nutritious lunch option, featuring roasted vegetables, protein-packed quinoa, and creamy tahini dressing.
*Prep Time:* 30 minutes

*Ingredients:*
- 1 cup cooked quinoa
- 2 cups mixed vegetables (such as bell peppers, carrots, zucchini)
- 2 tablespoons olive oil
- Salt and pepper to taste
- 1/4 cup tahini
- 2 tablespoons lemon juice
- 1 clove garlic, minced
- Water, as needed
- Fresh parsley for garnish

*Instructions:*
1. Preheat oven to 400°F (200°C) and line a baking sheet with parchment paper.
2. In a large bowl, toss mixed vegetables with olive oil, salt, and pepper until evenly coated.
3. Spread vegetables in a single layer on the prepared baking sheet.
4. Roast in the preheated oven for 20-25 minutes, or until vegetables are tender and caramelized.
5. In a small bowl, whisk together tahini, lemon juice, minced garlic, and water until smooth and creamy, adding water as needed to reach desired consistency.

6. To assemble the bowls, divide cooked quinoa and roasted vegetables among serving bowls.
7. Drizzle tahini dressing over the bowls and garnish with fresh parsley.
8. Serve immediately and enjoy this delicious and nutritious quinoa bowl.

*Nutritional Information:* (per serving)
- Calories: 350
- Protein: 10g
- Carbohydrates: 30g
- Fat: 20g
- Fiber: 8g

## **Egg Salad Lettuce Wraps with Dill**

*Introduction:* These egg salad lettuce wraps are a light and flavorful lunch option, featuring creamy egg salad flavored with fresh dill, wrapped in crisp lettuce leaves.
*Prep Time:* 15 minutes

*Ingredients:*
- 4 hard-boiled eggs, peeled and chopped
- 2 tablespoons mayonnaise
- 1 tablespoon Greek yogurt
- 1 tablespoon fresh dill, chopped
- 1 teaspoon Dijon mustard
- Salt and pepper to taste
- Lettuce leaves for wrapping
- Cherry tomatoes for garnish

*Instructions:*
1. In a bowl, combine chopped hard-boiled eggs, mayonnaise, Greek yogurt, chopped fresh dill, Dijon mustard, salt, and pepper.
2. Mix until well combined and creamy.
3. Spoon egg salad onto lettuce leaves.
4. Garnish with cherry tomatoes.
5. Roll up lettuce leaves and secure with toothpicks if needed.
6. Serve immediately and enjoy these light and delicious egg salad lettuce wraps.

*Nutritional Information:* (per serving)
- Calories: 180
- Protein: 12g
- Carbohydrates: 5g
- Fat: 12g
- Fiber: 2g

## Tomato Basil Soup with Whole Grain Crackers

*Introduction:* This tomato basil soup is a comforting and satisfying lunch option, perfect for cooler days, and pairs perfectly with whole grain crackers.
*Prep Time:* 25 minutes

*Ingredients:*
- 6 ripe tomatoes, diced
- 1 onion, chopped
- 2 cloves garlic, minced
- 4 cups vegetable broth
- 1/2 cup fresh basil leaves, chopped
- Salt and pepper to taste
- Whole grain crackers for serving

*Instructions:*
1. In a large pot, heat olive oil over medium heat.
2. Add chopped onion and minced garlic, and sauté until softened and fragrant.
3. Add diced tomatoes and cook until they start to break down.
4. Pour in vegetable broth and bring to a simmer.
5. Let the soup simmer for about 15-20 minutes, until the flavors meld together.
6. Stir in chopped basil leaves and season with salt and pepper to taste.
7. Using an immersion blender, blend the soup until smooth and creamy.
8. Serve hot, accompanied by whole grain crackers.

*Nutritional Information:* (per serving)
- Calories: 120
- Protein: 3g
- Carbohydrates: 20g
- Fat: 4g
- Fiber: 5g

## Sweet Potato and Black Bean Quesadilla with Salsa

*Introduction:* This sweet potato and black bean quesadilla is a flavorful and satisfying lunch option, filled with nutritious ingredients and served with salsa for dipping.
*Prep Time:* 30 minutes

*Ingredients:*
- 1 large sweet potato, peeled and diced
- 1 can black beans, drained and rinsed
- 1 teaspoon chili powder
- 1/2 teaspoon cumin
- 4 whole wheat tortillas

- 1 cup shredded cheese (cheddar or Mexican blend)
- Salsa for serving
- Guacamole or sour cream (optional)

*Instructions:*
1. Preheat oven to 400°F (200°C) and line a baking sheet with parchment paper.
2. In a bowl, toss diced sweet potato with chili powder and cumin until evenly coated.
3. Spread sweet potato on the prepared baking sheet and roast in the preheated oven for 20-25 minutes, or until tender and caramelized.
4. In a skillet over medium heat, warm one whole wheat tortilla.
5. Sprinkle shredded cheese evenly over the tortilla.
6. Spoon roasted sweet potato and black beans over half of the tortilla.
7. Fold the tortilla in half to cover the filling and press gently to seal.
8. Cook quesadilla for 2-3 minutes on each side, until cheese is melted and tortilla is golden brown.
9. Repeat with remaining tortillas and filling.
10. Serve quesadillas hot, accompanied by salsa and guacamole or sour cream if desired.

*Nutritional Information:* (per serving)
- Calories: 350
- Protein: 15g
- Carbohydrates: 45g
- Fat: 12g
- Fiber: 8g

## **Sushi Bowl with Brown Rice, Avocado, and Cucumber**

*Introduction:* This sushi bowl is a deconstructed version of sushi rolls, featuring brown rice, creamy avocado, crisp cucumber, and nori strips, perfect for a quick and satisfying lunch.
*Prep Time:* 20 minutes

*Ingredients:*
- 1 cup cooked brown rice
- 1/2 avocado, sliced
- 1/2 cucumber, julienned
- 1/4 cup shredded carrots
- 1/4 cup edamame, shelled
- 1 nori sheet, cut into strips
- Soy sauce or tamari for serving
- Pickled ginger and wasabi (optional)

*Instructions:*
1. Divide cooked brown rice among serving bowls.

2. Arrange sliced avocado, julienned cucumber, shredded carrots, and edamame over the rice.
3. Top with nori strips.
4. Serve with soy sauce or tamari on the side.
5. Add pickled ginger and wasabi if desired.
6. Enjoy this sushi bowl as a nutritious and satisfying lunch option.

*Nutritional Information:* (per serving)
- Calories: 300
- Protein: 8g
- Carbohydrates: 45g
- Fat: 12g
- Fiber: 10g

## **Turkey and Quinoa Stuffed Peppers**

*Introduction:* These turkey and quinoa stuffed peppers are a wholesome and flavorful lunch option, filled with lean protein, whole grains, and colorful vegetables.
*Prep Time:* 45 minutes

*Ingredients:*
- 4 large bell peppers, halved and seeds removed
- 1 pound lean ground turkey
- 1 cup cooked quinoa
- 1/2 onion, finely chopped
- 2 cloves garlic, minced
- 1 cup tomato sauce
- 1 teaspoon Italian seasoning
- Salt and pepper to taste
- Shredded mozzarella cheese for topping
- Fresh parsley for garnish

*Instructions:*
1. Preheat oven to 375°F (190°C) and grease a baking dish.
2. In a skillet over medium heat, cook ground turkey until browned.
3. Add chopped onion and minced garlic to the skillet and cook until softened.
4. Stir in cooked quinoa, tomato sauce, Italian seasoning, salt, and pepper.
5. Simmer for 5-7 minutes, allowing flavors to meld together.
6. Fill each halved bell pepper with the turkey and quinoa mixture.
7. Sprinkle shredded mozzarella cheese over the stuffed peppers.
8. Cover the baking dish with foil and bake in the preheated oven for 25-30 minutes, or until peppers are tender.
9. Remove foil and broil for an additional 2-3 minutes to melt and brown the cheese.
10. Garnish with fresh parsley before serving.

11. Enjoy these delicious and nutritious turkey and quinoa stuffed peppers.

*Nutritional Information:* (per serving, 1 stuffed pepper half)
- Calories: 280
- Protein: 25g
- Carbohydrates: 20g
- Fat: 10g
- Fiber: 5g

# Delicious Dinner Recipes

## Baked Salmon with Lemon and Dill

*Introduction:* This baked salmon recipe is simple yet flavorful, with zesty lemon and aromatic dill complementing the rich taste of the salmon.
*Prep Time:* 20 minutes

*Ingredients:*
- 4 salmon fillets
- 2 tablespoons olive oil
- 2 tablespoons lemon juice
- 2 cloves garlic, minced
- 1 tablespoon fresh dill, chopped
- Salt and pepper to taste
- Lemon slices for garnish

*Instructions:*
1. Preheat oven to 375°F (190°C) and line a baking dish with parchment paper.
2. Place salmon fillets in the prepared baking dish.
3. In a small bowl, whisk together olive oil, lemon juice, minced garlic, chopped dill, salt, and pepper.
4. Pour the mixture over the salmon fillets, ensuring they are evenly coated.
5. Place lemon slices on top of the salmon for extra flavor.
6. Bake in the preheated oven for 12-15 minutes, or until the salmon is cooked through and flakes easily with a fork.
7. Serve hot and enjoy this delicious baked salmon.

*Nutritional Information:* (per serving)
- Calories: 300
- Protein: 25g
- Carbohydrates: 2g
- Fat: 20g
- Fiber: 1g

## **Turkey Chili with Kidney Beans and Bell Peppers**

*Introduction:* This hearty turkey chili is loaded with lean protein, fiber-rich kidney beans, and colorful bell peppers, making it a comforting and nutritious dinner option.
*Prep Time:* 30 minutes

*Ingredients:*
- 1 pound ground turkey
- 1 onion, chopped
- 2 cloves garlic, minced
- 1 bell pepper, diced
- 1 can kidney beans, drained and rinsed
- 1 can diced tomatoes
- 2 cups chicken broth
- 2 tablespoons chili powder
- 1 teaspoon cumin
- Salt and pepper to taste
- Optional toppings: shredded cheese, sour cream, chopped cilantro

*Instructions:*
1. In a large pot, cook ground turkey over medium heat until browned.
2. Add chopped onion, minced garlic, and diced bell pepper to the pot, and cook until vegetables are softened.
3. Stir in kidney beans, diced tomatoes, chicken broth, chili powder, cumin, salt, and pepper.
4. Bring the chili to a simmer and let it cook for 20-25 minutes, stirring occasionally.
5. Adjust seasoning to taste if needed.
6. Serve hot, garnished with optional toppings if desired.
7. Enjoy this delicious and comforting turkey chili.

*Nutritional Information:* (per serving)
- Calories: 300
- Protein: 20g
- Carbohydrates: 25g
- Fat: 10g
- Fiber: 8g

## **Grilled Chicken Breast with Roasted Vegetables**

*Introduction:* This grilled chicken breast paired with roasted vegetables is a simple yet satisfying dinner option, perfect for a healthy and balanced meal.
*Prep Time:* 30 minutes

*Ingredients:*
- 4 boneless, skinless chicken breasts
- 2 tablespoons olive oil
- 2 cloves garlic, minced
- 1 teaspoon dried herbs (such as thyme, rosemary, or oregano)
- Salt and pepper to taste
- Assorted vegetables for roasting (such as bell peppers, zucchini, carrots, and red onions)
- Balsamic glaze for serving (optional)

*Instructions:*
1. Preheat grill to medium-high heat.
2. In a bowl, combine olive oil, minced garlic, dried herbs, salt, and pepper.
3. Brush the mixture over chicken breasts, coating them evenly.
4. Grill chicken breasts for 6-8 minutes per side, or until they are cooked through and no longer pink in the center.
5. While the chicken is grilling, prepare the vegetables for roasting by cutting them into bite-sized pieces.
6. Toss the vegetables with olive oil, salt, and pepper, and spread them out on a baking sheet.
7. Roast vegetables in a preheated oven at 400°F (200°C) for 20-25 minutes, or until they are tender and caramelized.
8. Serve grilled chicken breasts with roasted vegetables and drizzle with balsamic glaze if desired.
9. Enjoy this delicious and nutritious dinner.

*Nutritional Information:* (per serving)
- Calories: 350
- Protein: 30g
- Carbohydrates: 15g
- Fat: 15g
- Fiber: 5g

## Quinoa Stuffed Bell Peppers with Tomato Sauce

*Introduction:* These quinoa stuffed bell peppers are filled with a flavorful mixture of quinoa, vegetables, and spices, then baked until tender and topped with tangy tomato sauce.
*Prep Time:* 45 minutes

*Ingredients:*
- 4 large bell peppers, halved and seeds removed
- 1 cup cooked quinoa
- 1 onion, finely chopped
- 2 cloves garlic, minced
- 1 carrot, grated

- 1 zucchini, grated
- 1 cup diced tomatoes
- 1 teaspoon dried herbs (such as basil, oregano, or thyme)
- Salt and pepper to taste
- 1 cup tomato sauce
- Grated Parmesan cheese for garnish (optional)

*Instructions:*

1. Preheat oven to 375°F (190°C) and grease a baking dish.
2. In a skillet over medium heat, sauté chopped onion and minced garlic until softened.
3. Add grated carrot and zucchini to the skillet, and cook until vegetables are tender.
4. Stir in cooked quinoa, diced tomatoes, dried herbs, salt, and pepper, and cook for another 5 minutes, allowing flavors to meld together.
5. Fill each halved bell pepper with the quinoa mixture.
6. Place stuffed bell peppers in the prepared baking dish.
7. Pour tomato sauce over the stuffed peppers.
8. Cover the baking dish with foil and bake in the preheated oven for 25-30 minutes, or until the peppers are tender.
9. Remove foil and sprinkle grated Parmesan cheese over the peppers if desired.
10. Serve hot and enjoy these delicious quinoa stuffed bell peppers.

*Nutritional Information:* (per serving, 1 stuffed pepper half)
- Calories: 250
- Protein: 8g
- Carbohydrates: 35g
- Fat: 8g
- Fiber: 8g

## **Shrimp Stir-Fry with Broccoli and Snow Peas**

*Introduction:* This shrimp stir-fry is a quick and flavorful dinner option, featuring tender shrimp, crisp broccoli, and sweet snow peas, all tossed in a savory sauce.
*Prep Time:* 20 minutes

*Ingredients:*
- 1 pound shrimp, peeled and deveined
- 2 cups broccoli florets
- 1 cup snow peas, trimmed
- 2 cloves garlic, minced
- 1 tablespoon ginger, grated
- 2 tablespoons soy sauce
- 1 tablespoon oyster sauce
- 1 teaspoon sesame oil
- 1 tablespoon cornstarch

- 2 tablespoons water
- Cooked rice or noodles for serving
- Sesame seeds for garnish (optional)

*Instructions:*
1. In a small bowl, whisk together soy sauce, oyster sauce, sesame oil, cornstarch, and water to make the sauce.
2. Heat oil in a large skillet or wok over medium-high heat.
3. Add minced garlic and grated ginger to the skillet, and cook until fragrant.
4. Add shrimp to the skillet and cook until they turn pink and opaque.
5. Remove shrimp from the skillet and set aside.
6. In the same skillet, add broccoli florets and snow peas, and stir-fry until they are tender-crisp.
7. Return shrimp to the skillet and pour the sauce over the shrimp and vegetables.
8. Cook for another 2-3 minutes, or until the sauce thickens and coats the shrimp and vegetables.
9. Serve hot over cooked rice or noodles, garnished with sesame seeds if desired.
10. Enjoy this flavorful shrimp stir-fry for dinner.

*Nutritional Information:* (per serving)
- Calories: 250
- Protein: 25g
- Carbohydrates: 15g
- Fat: 8g
- Fiber: 5g

## **Baked Cod with Herbed Quinoa**

*Introduction:* This baked cod with herbed quinoa is a light and nutritious dinner option, featuring tender cod fillets seasoned with herbs and served alongside flavorful quinoa.
*Prep Time:* 30 minutes

*Ingredients:*
- 4 cod fillets
- 2 tablespoons olive oil
- 1 tablespoon lemon juice
- 2 cloves garlic, minced
- 1 teaspoon dried herbs (such as parsley, thyme, or dill)
- Salt and pepper to taste
- 1 cup quinoa
- 2 cups vegetable broth
- Fresh parsley for garnish

*Instructions:*
1. Preheat oven to 375°F (190°C) and line a baking dish with parchment paper.
2. Place cod fillets in the prepared baking dish.
3. In a small bowl, whisk together olive oil, lemon juice, minced garlic, dried herbs, salt, and pepper.
4. Pour the mixture over the cod fillets, coating them evenly.
5. Bake in the preheated oven for 15-20 minutes, or until the cod is cooked through and flakes easily with a fork.
6. While the cod is baking, rinse quinoa under cold water and drain well.
7. In a saucepan, bring vegetable broth to a boil.
8. Add quinoa to the saucepan, cover, and reduce heat to low.
9. Simmer quinoa for 15-20 minutes, or until the liquid is absorbed and quinoa is tender.
10. Fluff quinoa with a fork and stir in chopped fresh parsley.
11. Serve baked cod fillets over herbed quinoa.
12. Enjoy this light and flavorful dinner.

*Nutritional Information:* (per serving)
- Calories: 300
- Protein: 25g
- Carbohydrates: 20g
- Fat: 12g
- Fiber: 3g

## **Veggie and Lentil Curry with Brown Rice**

*Introduction:* This veggie and lentil curry is a hearty and flavorful dinner option, packed with protein-rich lentils, colorful vegetables, and aromatic spices, served over brown rice for a satisfying meal.
*Prep Time:* 45 minutes

*Ingredients:*
- 1 cup dry lentils, rinsed and drained
- 2 cups vegetable broth
- 1 onion, chopped
- 2 cloves garlic, minced
- 1 bell pepper, diced
- 1 zucchini, diced
- 1 carrot, diced
- 1 can diced tomatoes
- 1 can coconut milk
- 2 tablespoons curry powder
- 1 teaspoon turmeric
- Salt and pepper to taste
- Cooked brown rice for serving

- Fresh cilantro for garnish

*Instructions:*
1. In a large pot, combine dry lentils and vegetable broth.
2. Bring to a boil, then reduce heat to low and simmer for 20-25 minutes, or until lentils are tender.
3. In a separate skillet, heat olive oil over medium heat.
4. Add chopped onion and minced garlic to the skillet, and cook until softened.
5. Stir in diced bell pepper, zucchini, and carrot, and cook until vegetables are tender-crisp.
6. Add diced tomatoes, coconut milk, curry powder, turmeric, salt, and pepper to the skillet, and stir to combine.
7. Simmer curry sauce for 10-15 minutes, allowing flavors to meld together.
8. Once lentils are cooked, add them to the curry sauce and stir to combine.
9. Serve veggie and lentil curry over cooked brown rice.
10. Garnish with fresh cilantro before serving.
11. Enjoy this hearty and flavorful dinner.

*Nutritional Information:* (per serving)
- Calories: 350
- Protein: 15g
- Carbohydrates: 40g
- Fat: 15g
- Fiber: 10g

## Zucchini Noodles with Tomato Basil Sauce

*Introduction:* These zucchini noodles with tomato basil sauce are a light and refreshing dinner option, featuring spiralized zucchini noodles tossed in a vibrant tomato basil sauce.
*Prep Time:* 25 minutes

*Ingredients:*
- 4 medium zucchini
- 2 tablespoons olive oil
- 2 cloves garlic, minced
- 1 can crushed tomatoes
- 1/4 cup fresh basil leaves, chopped
- Salt and pepper to taste
- Grated Parmesan cheese for serving (optional)

*Instructions:*
1. Using a spiralizer, spiralize zucchini into noodles.
2. Heat olive oil in a skillet over medium heat.
3. Add minced garlic to the skillet and cook until fragrant.

4.  Pour crushed tomatoes into the skillet and simmer for 10-15 minutes, stirring occasionally.
5.  Stir in chopped fresh basil leaves, and season with salt and pepper to taste.
6.  While the sauce is simmering, heat a separate skillet over medium heat.
7.  Add zucchini noodles to the skillet and cook for 3-5 minutes, or until noodles are tender-crisp.
8.  Once zucchini noodles are cooked, divide them among serving plates.
9.  Spoon tomato basil sauce over the zucchini noodles.
10. Sprinkle grated Parmesan cheese over the noodles if desired.
11. Serve hot and enjoy this light and flavorful dinner.

*Nutritional Information:* (per serving)
- Calories: 150
- Protein: 5g
- Carbohydrates: 15g
- Fat: 10g
- Fiber: 5g

## Lemon Garlic Roasted Chicken with Steamed Green Beans

*Introduction:* This lemon garlic roasted chicken is tender and flavorful, with juicy chicken breasts marinated in zesty lemon and aromatic garlic, served with steamed green beans for a simple and satisfying dinner.
*Prep Time:* 40 minutes

*Ingredients:*
- 4 boneless, skinless chicken breasts
- 2 lemons, juiced and zest
- 4 cloves garlic, minced
- 2 tablespoons olive oil
- Salt and pepper to taste
- 1 pound green beans, trimmed
- Lemon slices for garnish

*Instructions:*
1.  In a bowl, whisk together lemon juice, lemon zest, minced garlic, olive oil, salt, and pepper to make the marinade.
2.  Place chicken breasts in a shallow dish and pour the marinade over them, turning to coat evenly.
3.  Cover and refrigerate chicken for at least 30 minutes, or up to 2 hours.
4.  Preheat oven to 375°F (190°C) and line a baking dish with parchment paper.
5.  Place marinated chicken breasts in the prepared baking dish.
6.  Bake in the preheated oven for 25-30 minutes, or until chicken is cooked through and juices run clear.

7. While the chicken is baking, steam green beans until they are tender-crisp.
8. Serve lemon garlic roasted chicken with steamed green beans.
9. Garnish with lemon slices before serving.
10. Enjoy this simple and flavorful dinner.

*Nutritional Information:* (per serving)
- Calories: 300
- Protein: 30g
- Carbohydrates: 10g
- Fat: 15g
- Fiber: 5g

## Turkey and Vegetable Skewers with Quinoa Pilaf

*Introduction:* These turkey and vegetable skewers are grilled to perfection, featuring tender turkey chunks and colorful vegetables, served with quinoa pilaf for a wholesome and satisfying dinner.
*Prep Time:* 45 minutes

*Ingredients:*
- 1 pound turkey breast, cut into chunks
- 2 bell peppers, cut into chunks
- 1 red onion, cut into chunks
- 1 zucchini, sliced
- 2 tablespoons olive oil
- 2 cloves garlic, minced
- 1 teaspoon dried herbs (such as rosemary, thyme, or oregano)
- Salt and pepper to taste
- Wooden skewers, soaked in water
- 1 cup quinoa
- 2 cups chicken broth
- Fresh parsley for garnish

*Instructions:*
1. In a bowl, combine turkey chunks, bell pepper chunks, onion chunks, zucchini slices, olive oil, minced garlic, dried herbs, salt, and pepper, and toss to coat evenly.
2. Thread marinated turkey and vegetables onto soaked wooden skewers.
3. Preheat grill to medium-high heat.
4. Grill skewers for 10-12 minutes, turning occasionally, until turkey is cooked through and vegetables are tender.
5. While the skewers are grilling, rinse quinoa under cold water and drain well.
6. In a saucepan, bring chicken broth to a boil.
7. Add quinoa to the saucepan, cover, and reduce heat to low.
8. Simmer quinoa for 15-20 minutes, or until the liquid is absorbed and quinoa is tender.

9.   Fluff quinoa with a fork and stir in chopped fresh parsley.
10.  Serve turkey and vegetable skewers with quinoa pilaf.
11.  Enjoy this wholesome and satisfying dinner.

*Nutritional Information:* (per serving)
- Calories: 350
- Protein: 25g
- Carbohydrates: 30g
- Fat: 15g
- Fiber: 5g

## **Stuffed Portobello Mushrooms with Spinach and Goat Cheese**

*Introduction:* These stuffed portobello mushrooms are filled with savory spinach and tangy goat cheese, baked until golden and bubbling for a delicious and satisfying dinner option.
*Prep Time:* 35 minutes

*Ingredients:*
- 4 large portobello mushrooms, stems removed
- 2 tablespoons olive oil
- 2 cloves garlic, minced
- 2 cups baby spinach, chopped
- 4 ounces goat cheese, crumbled
- Salt and pepper to taste
- Fresh parsley for garnish

*Instructions:*
1.   Preheat oven to 375°F (190°C) and line a baking sheet with parchment paper.
2.   Place portobello mushrooms on the prepared baking sheet, gill side up.
3.   In a skillet, heat olive oil over medium heat.
4.   Add minced garlic to the skillet and cook until fragrant.
5.   Add chopped baby spinach to the skillet and cook until wilted.
6.   Remove skillet from heat and stir in crumbled goat cheese until melted and combined.
7.   Season spinach and goat cheese mixture with salt and pepper to taste.
8.   Divide the spinach and goat cheese mixture among the portobello mushrooms, filling each cap evenly.
9.   Bake in the preheated oven for 20-25 minutes, or until mushrooms are tender and filling is golden and bubbling.
10.  Garnish with fresh parsley before serving.
11.  Enjoy these delicious stuffed portobello mushrooms for dinner.

*Nutritional Information:* (per serving)
- Calories: 200
- Protein: 10g

- Carbohydrates: 10g
- Fat: 15g
- Fiber: 3g

## Roasted Butternut Squash and Chickpea Salad

*Introduction:* This roasted butternut squash and chickpea salad is bursting with flavor and texture, featuring tender roasted squash, crisp chickpeas, and tangy feta cheese, all tossed in a zesty vinaigrette.
*Prep Time:* 40 minutes

*Ingredients:*
- 1 medium butternut squash, peeled, seeded, and diced
- 1 can chickpeas, drained and rinsed
- 2 tablespoons olive oil
- 1 teaspoon ground cumin
- 1 teaspoon paprika
- Salt and pepper to taste
- 4 cups mixed salad greens
- 1/2 cup crumbled feta cheese
- 1/4 cup dried cranberries
- Balsamic vinaigrette for serving

*Instructions:*
1. Preheat oven to 400°F (200°C) and line a baking sheet with parchment paper.
2. In a bowl, toss diced butternut squash and chickpeas with olive oil, ground cumin, paprika, salt, and pepper until evenly coated.
3. Spread the butternut squash and chickpeas in a single layer on the prepared baking sheet.
4. Roast in the preheated oven for 25-30 minutes, or until squash is tender and chickpeas are crispy.
5. In a large salad bowl, combine mixed greens, roasted butternut squash, chickpeas, crumbled feta cheese, and dried cranberries.
6. Drizzle with balsamic vinaigrette and toss to coat evenly.
7. Serve immediately and enjoy this delicious roasted butternut squash and chickpea salad.

*Nutritional Information:* (per serving)
- Calories: 250
- Protein: 8g
- Carbohydrates: 30g
- Fat: 12g
- Fiber: 8g

## **Veggie Stir-Fry with Tofu and Brown Rice**

*Introduction:* This veggie stir-fry with tofu and brown rice is a nutritious and flavorful dinner option, featuring colorful vegetables, protein-rich tofu, and wholesome brown rice, all tossed in a savory sauce.
*Prep Time:* 35 minutes

*Ingredients:*
- 1 block firm tofu, pressed and cubed
- 2 tablespoons soy sauce
- 1 tablespoon sesame oil
- 2 cloves garlic, minced
- 1 tablespoon ginger, grated
- Assorted vegetables (such as bell peppers, broccoli, carrots, and snow peas), sliced
- Cooked brown rice for serving
- Sesame seeds for garnish

*Instructions:*
1. In a bowl, toss cubed tofu with soy sauce and sesame oil until evenly coated.
2. Heat a skillet or wok over medium-high heat.
3. Add minced garlic and grated ginger to the skillet, and cook until fragrant.
4. Add marinated tofu to the skillet and cook until golden brown and crispy on all sides.
5. Remove tofu from the skillet and set aside.
6. In the same skillet, add assorted vegetables and stir-fry until they are tender-crisp.
7. Return tofu to the skillet and toss with vegetables.
8. Serve veggie stir-fry over cooked brown rice.
9. Garnish with sesame seeds before serving.
10. Enjoy this nutritious and flavorful dinner.

*Nutritional Information:* (per serving)
- Calories: 300
- Protein: 15g
- Carbohydrates: 35g
- Fat: 12g
- Fiber: 8g

## **Baked Chicken Thighs with Sweet Potatoes and Brussels Sprouts**

*Introduction:* These baked chicken thighs with sweet potatoes and Brussels sprouts are a comforting and wholesome dinner option, featuring tender chicken thighs and roasted vegetables seasoned with herbs and spices.
*Prep Time:* 50 minutes

*Ingredients:*
- 4 chicken thighs, bone-in and skin-on
- 2 sweet potatoes, peeled and diced
- 1 pound Brussels sprouts, trimmed and halved
- 2 tablespoons olive oil
- 2 cloves garlic, minced
- 1 teaspoon dried herbs (such as rosemary, thyme, or sage)
- Salt and pepper to taste
- Fresh parsley for garnish

*Instructions:*
1. Preheat oven to 400°F (200°C) and line a baking sheet with parchment paper.
2. Place chicken thighs on one side of the prepared baking sheet.
3. In a bowl, toss diced sweet potatoes and halved Brussels sprouts with olive oil, minced garlic, dried herbs, salt, and pepper until evenly coated.
4. Spread the sweet potatoes and Brussels sprouts on the other side of the baking sheet.
5. Bake in the preheated oven for 30-35 minutes, or until chicken thighs are cooked through and vegetables are tender and caramelized.
6. Remove from the oven and let rest for 5 minutes.
7. Serve baked chicken thighs with sweet potatoes and Brussels sprouts.
8. Garnish with fresh parsley before serving.
9. Enjoy this comforting and wholesome dinner.

*Nutritional Information:* (per serving)
- Calories: 400
- Protein: 25g
- Carbohydrates: 30g
- Fat: 20g
- Fiber: 8g

## **Spaghetti Squash with Garlic and Parmesan**

*Introduction:* This spaghetti squash with garlic and Parmesan is a light and flavorful dinner option, featuring tender spaghetti squash strands tossed in a garlic-infused olive oil and topped with grated Parmesan cheese.
*Prep Time:* 40 minutes

*Ingredients:*
- 1 large spaghetti squash
- 2 tablespoons olive oil
- 4 cloves garlic, minced
- Salt and pepper to taste
- Grated Parmesan cheese for serving
- Fresh parsley for garnish

*Instructions:*
1. Preheat oven to 400°F (200°C) and line a baking sheet with parchment paper.
2. Cut spaghetti squash in half lengthwise and scoop out the seeds.
3. Place squash halves cut side down on the prepared baking sheet.
4. Bake in the preheated oven for 30-35 minutes, or until squash is tender and easily pierced with a fork.
5. While the squash is baking, heat olive oil in a skillet over medium heat.
6. Add minced garlic to the skillet and cook until fragrant, about 1 minute.
7. Using a fork, scrape the flesh of the cooked spaghetti squash to create strands.
8. Add spaghetti squash strands to the skillet with garlic-infused olive oil.
9. Toss until squash is evenly coated with garlic oil.
10. Season with salt and pepper to taste.
11. Serve spaghetti squash with grated Parmesan cheese and fresh parsley.
12. Enjoy this light and flavorful dinner.

*Nutritional Information:* (per serving)
- Calories: 200
- Protein: 5g
- Carbohydrates: 25g
- Fat: 10g
- Fiber: 5g

# Healthy Snack Recipes

## Sliced Apple with Almond Butter

*Introduction:* This simple and nutritious snack pairs crisp apple slices with creamy almond butter for a satisfying and energizing treat.
*Prep Time:* 5 minutes

*Ingredients:*
- 1 apple, sliced
- 2 tablespoons almond butter

*Instructions:*
1. Wash and slice the apple into thin slices.
2. Spread almond butter on each apple slice.
3. Arrange on a plate and enjoy this delicious snack.

*Nutritional Information:* (per serving)
- Calories: 150
- Protein: 3g
- Carbohydrates: 20g
- Fat: 8g

- Fiber: 5g

## **Carrot Sticks with Hummus**

*Introduction:* Crunchy carrot sticks paired with creamy hummus make for a nutritious and satisfying snack, perfect for any time of day.
*Prep Time:* 10 minutes

*Ingredients:*
- 2 carrots, peeled and cut into sticks
- 1/4 cup hummus
- *Instructions:*
1. Wash, peel, and cut carrots into sticks.
2. Serve carrot sticks with hummus for dipping.
3. Enjoy this refreshing and healthy snack.

*Nutritional Information:* (per serving)
- Calories: 100
- Protein: 3g
- Carbohydrates: 10g
- Fat: 6g
- Fiber: 4g

## **Greek Yogurt with Honey and Walnuts**

*Introduction:* Creamy Greek yogurt drizzled with honey and sprinkled with crunchy walnuts creates a delicious and satisfying snack that's rich in protein and healthy fats.
*Prep Time:* 5 minutes

*Ingredients:*
- 1/2 cup Greek yogurt
- 1 tablespoon honey
- 2 tablespoons chopped walnuts

*Instructions:*
1. Spoon Greek yogurt into a bowl.
2. Drizzle honey over the yogurt.
3. Sprinkle chopped walnuts on top.
4. Enjoy this indulgent yet healthy snack.

*Nutritional Information:* (per serving)
- Calories: 200
- Protein: 15g
- Carbohydrates: 15g

- Fat: 10g
- Fiber: 2g

## Rice Cake with Avocado and Tomato Slices

*Introduction:* This rice cake topped with creamy avocado and fresh tomato slices is a light and satisfying snack that's perfect for a quick pick-me-up.
*Prep Time:* 5 minutes

*Ingredients:*
- 1 rice cake
- 1/2 avocado, sliced
- 1/2 tomato, sliced

*Instructions:*
1. Place a rice cake on a plate.
2. Arrange avocado slices on top of the rice cake.
3. Top with tomato slices.
4. Enjoy this simple and nutritious snack.

*Nutritional Information:* (per serving)
- Calories: 120
- Protein: 2g
- Carbohydrates: 15g
- Fat: 7g
- Fiber: 4g

## Celery Sticks with Peanut Butter

*Introduction:* Crunchy celery sticks paired with creamy peanut butter create a classic and satisfying snack that's perfect for satisfying cravings and providing lasting energy.
*Prep Time:* 5 minutes

*Ingredients:*
- 2 celery stalks, cut into sticks
- 2 tablespoons peanut butter

*Instructions:*
1. Wash and cut celery stalks into sticks.
2. Spread peanut butter on each celery stick.
3. Arrange on a plate and enjoy this delicious and nutritious snack.

*Nutritional Information:* (per serving)
- Calories: 150

- Protein: 4g
- Carbohydrates: 8g
- Fat: 12g
- Fiber: 4g

## Edamame Beans with Sea Salt

*Introduction:* Edamame beans sprinkled with sea salt make for a flavorful and protein-rich snack that's perfect for munching on between meals.
*Prep Time:* 10 minutes

*Ingredients:*
- 1 cup edamame beans, cooked and shelled
- Sea salt to taste

*Instructions:*
1. Cook edamame beans according to package instructions and shell them if necessary.
2. Sprinkle edamame beans with sea salt to taste.
3. Serve and enjoy this tasty and nutritious snack.

*Nutritional Information:* (per serving)
- Calories: 100
- Protein: 9g
- Carbohydrates: 8g
- Fat: 3g
- Fiber: 4g

## Roasted Chickpeas with Rosemary

*Introduction:* These crunchy roasted chickpeas seasoned with aromatic rosemary make for a satisfying and flavorful snack that's high in protein and fiber.
*Prep Time:* 45 minutes

*Ingredients:*
- 1 can chickpeas, drained and rinsed
- 1 tablespoon olive oil
- 1 teaspoon dried rosemary
- Salt and pepper to taste

*Instructions:*
1. Preheat oven to 400°F (200°C) and line a baking sheet with parchment paper.
2. Pat chickpeas dry with a paper towel and remove any loose skins.
3. In a bowl, toss chickpeas with olive oil, dried rosemary, salt, and pepper until evenly coated.

4. Spread chickpeas in a single layer on the prepared baking sheet.
5. Bake in the preheated oven for 30-40 minutes, or until chickpeas are golden and crispy.
6. Let cool before serving.
7. Enjoy these delicious roasted chickpeas as a healthy snack.

*Nutritional Information:* (per serving)
- Calories: 150
- Protein: 7g
- Carbohydrates: 20g
- Fat: 5g
- Fiber: 6g

## Whole Grain Crackers with Goat Cheese

*Introduction:* Whole grain crackers paired with creamy goat cheese make for a satisfying and flavorful snack that's perfect for satisfying cravings while being mindful of portion sizes.
*Prep Time:* 5 minutes

*Ingredients:*
- 4 whole grain crackers
- 2 ounces goat cheese

*Instructions:*
1. Spread goat cheese on each whole grain cracker.
2. Serve and enjoy this delicious and satisfying snack.

*Nutritional Information:* (per serving)
- Calories: 200
- Protein: 8g
- Carbohydrates: 20g
- Fat: 10g
- Fiber: 4g

## Bell Pepper Strips with Guacamole

*Introduction:* Crisp bell pepper strips paired with creamy guacamole create a colorful and satisfying snack that's packed with flavor and nutrients.
*Prep Time:* 10 minutes

*Ingredients:*
- 2 bell peppers, sliced into strips
- 1 ripe avocado
- 1/2 lime, juiced
- Salt and pepper to taste

*Instructions:*
1. Slice bell peppers into strips.
2. In a bowl, mash ripe avocado with lime juice, salt, and pepper to make guacamole.
3. Serve bell pepper strips with guacamole for dipping.
4. Enjoy this vibrant and nutritious snack.

*Nutritional Information:* (per serving)
- Calories: 150
- Protein: 3g
- Carbohydrates: 10g
- Fat: 12g
- Fiber: 6g

## **Almonds and Dried Cranberries**

*Introduction:* A handful of almonds paired with sweet dried cranberries makes for a satisfying and nutritious snack that's perfect for satisfying hunger between meals, while being mindful of portion sizes.
*Prep Time:* 5 minutes

*Ingredients:*
- 1/4 cup almonds
- 2 tablespoons dried cranberries

*Instructions:*
1. Combine almonds and dried cranberries in a small bowl.
2. Toss to mix evenly.
3. Enjoy this simple and satisfying snack.

*Nutritional Information:* (per serving)
- Calories: 200
- Protein: 5g
- Carbohydrates: 15g
- Fat: 12g
- Fiber: 4g

## **Banana with Peanut Butter**

*Introduction:* Creamy peanut butter spread on ripe banana slices makes for a delicious and satisfying snack that's perfect for a quick energy boost.
*Prep Time:* 5 minutes

*Ingredients:*
- 1 ripe banana, sliced

- 2 tablespoons peanut butter

*Instructions:*
1. Slice ripe banana into rounds.
2. Spread peanut butter on each banana slice.
3. Enjoy this delicious and nutritious snack.

*Nutritional Information:* (per serving)
- Calories: 200
- Protein: 4g
- Carbohydrates: 25g
- Fat: 10g
- Fiber: 4g

## Cucumber Slices with Hummus

*Introduction:* Cool cucumber slices paired with creamy hummus create a refreshing and satisfying snack that's perfect for keeping hunger at bay between meals.
*Prep Time:* 10 minutes

*Ingredients:*
- 1 cucumber, sliced
- 1/4 cup hummus

*Instructions:*
1. Wash and slice cucumber into rounds.
2. Serve cucumber slices with hummus for dipping.
3. Enjoy this light and healthy snack.

*Nutritional Information:* (per serving)
- Calories: 100
- Protein: 3g
- Carbohydrates: 10g
- Fat: 6g
- Fiber: 4g

## Whole Wheat Pita with Tzatziki

*Introduction:* Whole wheat pita bread served with creamy tzatziki sauce makes for a flavorful and satisfying snack that's perfect for any time of day.
*Prep Time:* 10 minutes

*Ingredients:*
- 1 whole wheat pita bread, cut into triangles

  - 1/4 cup tzatziki sauce

*Instructions:*
1. Cut whole wheat pita bread into triangles.
2. Serve pita triangles with tzatziki sauce for dipping.
3. Enjoy this delicious and satisfying snack.

*Nutritional Information:* (per serving)
- Calories: 150
- Protein: 5g
- Carbohydrates: 20g
- Fat: 6g
- Fiber: 3g

## Avocado with Lime and Sea Salt

*Introduction:* Creamy avocado slices seasoned with tangy lime juice and sea salt make for a simple yet satisfying snack that's packed with healthy fats and flavor.
*Prep Time:* 5 minutes

*Ingredients:*
- 1 ripe avocado, sliced
- 1/2 lime, juiced
- Sea salt to taste

*Instructions:*
1. Slice ripe avocado and arrange on a plate.
2. Squeeze lime juice over avocado slices.
3. Sprinkle sea salt to taste.
4. Enjoy this delicious and nutritious snack.

*Nutritional Information:* (per serving)
- Calories: 200
- Protein: 3g
- Carbohydrates: 10g
- Fat: 18g
- Fiber: 7g

## Baked Kale Chips

*Introduction:* Crispy baked kale chips seasoned with aromatic spices make for a flavorful and nutritious snack that's perfect for munching on guilt-free.
*Prep Time:* 20 minutes

*Ingredients:*
- 1 bunch kale, washed and dried
- 1 tablespoon olive oil
- 1 teaspoon garlic powder
- 1/2 teaspoon paprika
- Salt to taste

*Instructions:*
1. Preheat oven to 350°F (175°C) and line a baking sheet with parchment paper.
2. Remove kale leaves from stems and tear into bite-sized pieces.
3. In a bowl, toss kale pieces with olive oil, garlic powder, paprika, and salt until evenly coated.
4. Spread kale pieces in a single layer on the prepared baking sheet.
5. Bake in the preheated oven for 10-15 minutes, or until kale is crispy but not burnt.
6. Let cool before serving.
7. Enjoy these crispy baked kale chips as a healthy and delicious snack.

*Nutritional Information:* (per serving)
- Calories: 100
- Protein: 5g
- Carbohydrates: 10g
- Fat: 6g
- Fiber: 5g

# Delicious Dessert Recipes

## Baked Apples with Cinnamon and Honey

*Introduction:* Baked apples with cinnamon and honey are a comforting and wholesome dessert, perfect for cooler evenings and simple indulgence.
*Prep Time:* 40 minutes

*Ingredients:*
- 4 apples, cored
- 2 tablespoons honey
- 1 teaspoon ground cinnamon
- 1/4 cup water

*Instructions:*
1. Preheat oven to 375°F (190°C) and grease a baking dish.
2. Place cored apples in the baking dish.
3. In a small bowl, mix honey and cinnamon.
4. Fill the center of each apple with the honey-cinnamon mixture.
5. Pour water into the baking dish.

6. Bake apples for 30-35 minutes, or until tender.
7. Serve warm and enjoy these delicious baked apples.

*Nutritional Information:* (per serving)
- Calories: 150
- Protein: 1g
- Carbohydrates: 40g
- Fat: 0g
- Fiber: 5g

## Chia Seed Pudding with Berries

*Introduction:* Chia seed pudding with berries is a nutritious and satisfying dessert option, packed with omega-3 fatty acids, fiber, and antioxidants.
*Prep Time:* 5 minutes (plus chilling time)

*Ingredients:*
- 1/4 cup chia seeds
- 1 cup almond milk (or any milk of choice)
- 1 tablespoon honey or maple syrup (optional)
- Mixed berries for topping

*Instructions:*
1. In a bowl, whisk together chia seeds, almond milk, and honey or maple syrup (if using).
2. Cover and refrigerate for at least 2 hours or overnight, until the pudding has thickened.
3. Stir the pudding before serving to ensure the chia seeds are evenly distributed.
4. Top with mixed berries before serving.
5. Enjoy this nutritious and delicious chia seed pudding.

*Nutritional Information:* (per serving)
- Calories: 150
- Protein: 5g
- Carbohydrates: 20g
- Fat: 6g
- Fiber: 8g

## Mixed Fruit Salad with Mint

*Introduction:* A mixed fruit salad with mint is a refreshing and vibrant dessert option, perfect for summer gatherings or as a light and healthy treat.
*Prep Time:* 15 minutes

*Ingredients:*
- Assorted fruits (such as strawberries, blueberries, kiwi, pineapple, grapes, and oranges), diced or sliced
- Fresh mint leaves, chopped
- Honey or maple syrup (optional)

*Instructions:*
1. Wash and prepare the fruits as needed, cutting them into bite-sized pieces.
2. In a large bowl, combine the diced or sliced fruits.
3. Add chopped mint leaves and gently toss to combine.
4. Drizzle with honey or maple syrup if desired.
5. Serve chilled and enjoy this refreshing mixed fruit salad.

*Nutritional Information:* (per serving)
- Calories: varies based on fruit selection
- Protein: varies
- Carbohydrates: varies
- Fat: varies
- Fiber: varies

## Mango Sorbet with Coconut Flakes

*Introduction:* Mango sorbet with coconut flakes is a tropical and refreshing dessert option, perfect for cooling down on hot summer days.
*Prep Time:* 10 minutes (plus freezing time)

*Ingredients:*
- 2 ripe mangoes, peeled and diced
- 1 tablespoon honey or maple syrup (optional)
- 1/4 cup coconut flakes

*Instructions:*
1. Place diced mangoes in a blender or food processor.
2. Add honey or maple syrup if additional sweetness is desired.
3. Blend until smooth and creamy.
4. Transfer the mango puree to a shallow dish or ice cube tray.
5. Freeze for 4-6 hours, or until firm.
6. Before serving, let the sorbet sit at room temperature for a few minutes to soften slightly.
7. Scoop sorbet into bowls or cones and sprinkle with coconut flakes.
8. Enjoy this tropical and refreshing mango sorbet.

*Nutritional Information:* (per serving)
- Calories: 100
- Protein: 1g

- Carbohydrates: 25g
- Fat: 2g
- Fiber: 3g

## Strawberry Banana Frozen Yogurt

*Introduction:* Strawberry banana frozen yogurt is a creamy and delicious dessert option, combining the natural sweetness of strawberries and bananas with tangy yogurt.
*Prep Time:* 10 minutes (plus freezing time)

*Ingredients:*
- 2 cups frozen strawberries
- 2 ripe bananas, sliced and frozen
- 1 cup Greek yogurt
- 2 tablespoons honey or maple syrup (optional)

*Instructions:*
1. In a blender or food processor, combine frozen strawberries, frozen bananas, Greek yogurt, and honey or maple syrup if desired.
2. Blend until smooth and creamy, scraping down the sides as needed.
3. Transfer the mixture to a shallow dish and freeze for 2-3 hours, or until firm.
4. Before serving, let the frozen yogurt sit at room temperature for a few minutes to soften slightly.
5. Scoop into bowls or cones and enjoy this creamy and refreshing dessert.

*Nutritional Information:* (per serving)
- Calories: 150
- Protein: 5g
- Carbohydrates: 30g
- Fat: 1g
- Fiber: 5g

## Coconut Rice Pudding with Mango

*Introduction:* Coconut rice pudding with mango is a creamy and tropical dessert option, combining aromatic coconut milk-infused rice with sweet and juicy mango chunks.
*Prep Time:* 45 minutes

*Ingredients:*
- 1 cup jasmine rice
- 1 can (13.5 oz) coconut milk
- 1/4 cup sugar
- 1 teaspoon vanilla extract
- 1 ripe mango, peeled and diced

- Toasted coconut flakes for garnish

*Instructions:*
1. Rinse jasmine rice under cold water until the water runs clear.
2. In a saucepan, combine rinsed rice, coconut milk, sugar, and vanilla extract.
3. Bring the mixture to a boil, then reduce heat to low and simmer for 30-35 minutes, stirring occasionally, until the rice is cooked and the mixture thickens.
4. Remove from heat and let the rice pudding cool slightly.
5. Serve the rice pudding in bowls, topped with diced mango and toasted coconut flakes.
6. Enjoy this creamy and indulgent coconut rice pudding with mango.

*Nutritional Information:* (per serving)
- Calories: 300
- Protein: 4g
- Carbohydrates: 50g
- Fat: 10g
- Fiber: 2g

## **Lemon Blueberry Yogurt Bark**

*Introduction:* Lemon blueberry yogurt bark is a refreshing and nutritious dessert option, featuring creamy yogurt infused with tangy lemon and sweet blueberries, frozen into a delightful treat.
*Prep Time:* 10 minutes (plus freezing time)

*Ingredients:*
- 2 cups Greek yogurt
- Zest of 1 lemon
- 2 tablespoons honey or maple syrup
- 1/2 cup fresh blueberries

*Instructions:*
1. In a bowl, combine Greek yogurt, lemon zest, and honey or maple syrup.
2. Line a baking sheet with parchment paper.
3. Spread the yogurt mixture evenly onto the parchment paper.
4. Sprinkle fresh blueberries over the yogurt mixture.
5. Place the baking sheet in the freezer and freeze for 2-3 hours, or until firm.
6. Once frozen, break the yogurt bark into pieces.
7. Serve immediately and enjoy this refreshing lemon blueberry yogurt bark.

*Nutritional Information:* (per serving)
- Calories: 100
- Protein: 8g
- Carbohydrates: 15g

- Fat: 2g
- Fiber: 1g

## **Frozen Banana Bites with Dark Chocolate**

*Introduction:* Frozen banana bites with dark chocolate are a delicious and satisfying dessert option, combining creamy bananas with rich and indulgent dark chocolate, perfect for a sweet treat.
*Prep Time:* 30 minutes (plus freezing time)

*Ingredients:*
- 2 ripe bananas, peeled and sliced into rounds
- 1/2 cup dark chocolate chips
- 1 tablespoon coconut oil
- Optional toppings: chopped nuts, shredded coconut, sea salt

*Instructions:*
1. Place banana slices on a parchment-lined baking sheet.
2. Freeze banana slices for at least 30 minutes, or until firm.
3. In a microwave-safe bowl, combine dark chocolate chips and coconut oil.
4. Microwave in 30-second intervals, stirring in between, until chocolate is melted and smooth.
5. Dip frozen banana slices into the melted chocolate, coating them halfway.
6. Place chocolate-coated banana slices back on the parchment-lined baking sheet.
7. Sprinkle optional toppings over the chocolate-coated banana slices.
8. Return the baking sheet to the freezer and freeze for an additional 30 minutes, or until the chocolate is set.
9. Serve and enjoy these delicious frozen banana bites with dark chocolate.

*Nutritional Information:* (per serving)
- Calories: 150
- Protein: 2g
- Carbohydrates: 20g
- Fat: 8g
- Fiber: 3g

## **Baked Pears with Maple Syrup and Walnuts**

*Introduction:* Baked pears with maple syrup and walnuts are a simple and elegant dessert option, featuring tender and caramelized pears topped with sweet maple syrup and crunchy walnuts.
*Prep Time:* 30 minutes

*Ingredients:*
- 4 ripe pears, halved and cored
- 1/4 cup maple syrup
- 1/4 cup chopped walnuts
- Ground cinnamon for sprinkling

*Instructions:*
1. Preheat oven to 375°F (190°C) and grease a baking dish.
2. Place pear halves, cut side up, in the baking dish.
3. Drizzle maple syrup over the pear halves.
4. Sprinkle chopped walnuts over the pears.
5. Lightly sprinkle ground cinnamon over the top.
6. Bake for 20-25 minutes, or until pears are tender and caramelized.
7. Serve warm and enjoy these delightful baked pears.

*Nutritional Information:* (per serving)
- Calories: 200
- Protein: 2g
- Carbohydrates: 40g
- Fat: 5g
- Fiber: 6g

## **Greek Yogurt Cheesecake with Berry Compote**

*Introduction:* Greek yogurt cheesecake with berry compote is a lighter and healthier twist on the classic cheesecake, featuring creamy Greek yogurt and a vibrant berry compote topping.
*Prep Time:* 1 hour (plus chilling time)

*Ingredients:*
For the crust:
- 1 1/2 cups graham cracker crumbs
- 1/4 cup melted butter

For the filling:
- 2 cups Greek yogurt
- 1/2 cup cream cheese
- 1/2 cup sugar
- 2 eggs
- 1 teaspoon vanilla extract

For the berry compote:
- 2 cups mixed berries (such as strawberries, blueberries, raspberries)
- 1/4 cup sugar
- 1 tablespoon lemon juice

*Instructions:*

1. Preheat oven to 325°F (160°C) and grease a 9-inch springform pan.
2. In a bowl, combine graham cracker crumbs and melted butter until evenly moistened.
3. Press the crumb mixture into the bottom of the prepared springform pan.
4. In a separate bowl, beat Greek yogurt, cream cheese, sugar, eggs, and vanilla extract until smooth and creamy.
5. Pour the filling over the crust in the springform pan.
6. Bake for 45-50 minutes, or until the center is set and edges are lightly golden.
7. Let the cheesecake cool completely, then refrigerate for at least 4 hours or overnight.
8. In a saucepan, combine mixed berries, sugar, and lemon juice.
9. Cook over medium heat, stirring occasionally, until the berries break down and the mixture thickens into a compote.
10. Let the berry compote cool completely before serving with the cheesecake.
11. Slice and serve this delightful Greek yogurt cheesecake with berry compote.

*Nutritional Information:* (per serving)
- Calories: 300
- Protein: 10g
- Carbohydrates: 30g
- Fat: 15g
- Fiber: 3g

## **Pineapple Coconut Ice Pops**

*Introduction:* Pineapple coconut ice pops are a tropical and refreshing dessert option, featuring juicy pineapple chunks and creamy coconut milk frozen into delightful ice pops.
*Prep Time:* 10 minutes (plus freezing time)

*Ingredients:*
- 2 cups pineapple chunks
- 1 can (13.5 oz) coconut milk
- 2 tablespoons honey or maple syrup (optional)
- Ice pop molds
- Ice pop sticks

*Instructions:*

1. In a blender or food processor, combine pineapple chunks, coconut milk, and honey or maple syrup if desired.
2. Blend until smooth and creamy.
3. Pour the mixture into ice pop molds, leaving a little space at the top for expansion.
4. Insert ice pop sticks into the molds.
5. Freeze for 4-6 hours, or until completely frozen.
6. To release the ice pops, run the molds under warm water for a few seconds.
7. Serve and enjoy these tropical pineapple coconut ice pops.

*Nutritional Information:* (per serving)
- Calories: 150
- Protein: 2g
- Carbohydrates: 20g
- Fat: 8g
- Fiber: 2g

## **Baked Peaches with Oat Crumble**

*Introduction:* Baked peaches with oat crumble are a comforting and wholesome dessert option, featuring ripe peaches topped with a crunchy oat topping, perfect for any occasion.
*Prep Time:* 30 minutes

*Ingredients:*
For the peaches:
- 4 ripe peaches, halved and pitted
- 2 tablespoons honey

For the oat crumble:
- 1/2 cup old-fashioned oats
- 1/4 cup flour (all-purpose or whole wheat)
- 1/4 cup brown sugar
- 1/4 teaspoon ground cinnamon
- 1/4 cup melted butter

*Instructions:*
1. Preheat oven to 375°F (190°C) and grease a baking dish.
2. Place peach halves, cut side up, in the baking dish.
3. Drizzle honey over the peach halves.
4. In a bowl, combine oats, flour, brown sugar, cinnamon, and melted butter until crumbly.
5. Spoon the oat crumble mixture evenly over the peach halves.
6. Bake for 25-30 minutes, or until the peaches are tender and the oat topping is golden brown.
7. Serve warm and enjoy these delicious baked peaches with oat crumble.

*Nutritional Information:* (per serving)
- Calories: 200
- Protein: 3g
- Carbohydrates: 30g
- Fat: 8g
- Fiber: 4g

## Raspberry Chia Jam with Whole Grain Toast

*Introduction:* Raspberry chia jam with whole grain toast is a nutritious and delicious dessert option, featuring homemade jam made with fresh raspberries and chia seeds, served on whole grain toast.
*Prep Time:* 20 minutes (plus chilling time)

*Ingredients:*
- 2 cups fresh raspberries
- 2 tablespoons chia seeds
- 2 tablespoons honey or maple syrup
- Whole grain bread, toasted

*Instructions:*
1. In a saucepan, heat raspberries over medium heat, stirring occasionally, until they begin to break down and release their juices.
2. Mash the raspberries with a fork or potato masher.
3. Stir in chia seeds and honey or maple syrup.
4. Reduce heat to low and simmer for 10-15 minutes, stirring frequently, until the jam thickens.
5. Remove from heat and let the jam cool completely.
6. Spread raspberry chia jam on toasted whole grain bread slices.
7. Serve and enjoy this nutritious and delicious raspberry chia jam with whole grain toast.

*Nutritional Information:* (per serving)
- Calories: 150
- Protein: 3g
- Carbohydrates: 25g
- Fat: 5g
- Fiber: 6g

## Apricot and Almond Energy Bites

*Introduction:* Apricot and almond energy bites are a nutritious and portable dessert option, featuring dried apricots, almonds, and oats, rolled into bite-sized snacks for a quick burst of energy.
*Prep Time:* 15 minutes

*Ingredients:*
- 1 cup dried apricots
- 1/2 cup almonds
- 1/2 cup rolled oats
- 2 tablespoons honey or maple syrup
- 1/2 teaspoon vanilla extract

- Pinch of salt

*Instructions:*
1. In a food processor, pulse dried apricots, almonds, rolled oats, honey or maple syrup, vanilla extract, and salt until the mixture comes together and forms a sticky dough.
2. Roll the dough into small balls using your hands.
3. Place the energy bites on a parchment-lined baking sheet.
4. Refrigerate for at least 30 minutes to firm up.
5. Once firm, transfer the energy bites to an airtight container and store in the refrigerator.
6. Enjoy these nutritious and delicious apricot and almond energy bites as a sweet and satisfying dessert.

*Nutritional Information:* (per serving)
- Calories: 100
- Protein: 3g
- Carbohydrates: 15g
- Fat: 5g
- Fiber: 2g

## Coconut Mango Rice Cake

*Introduction:* Coconut mango rice cake is a tropical and flavorful dessert option, featuring aromatic coconut-infused rice topped with sweet and juicy mango slices, perfect for satisfying sweet cravings.
*Prep Time:* 45 minutes

*Ingredients:*
- 1 cup jasmine rice
- 1 can (13.5 oz) coconut milk
- 1/4 cup sugar
- 1 teaspoon vanilla extract
- 2 ripe mangoes, peeled and sliced
- Toasted coconut flakes for garnish

*Instructions:*
1. Rinse jasmine rice under cold water until the water runs clear.
2. In a saucepan, combine rinsed rice, coconut milk, sugar, and vanilla extract.
3. Bring the mixture to a boil, then reduce heat to low and simmer for 20-25 minutes, stirring occasionally, until the rice is cooked and the mixture thickens.
4. Remove from heat and let the coconut rice cool slightly.
5. Transfer the coconut rice to serving bowls or plates.
6. Top with sliced mangoes and sprinkle with toasted coconut flakes.
7. Serve and enjoy this delicious coconut mango rice cake.

*Nutritional Information:* (per serving)
- Calories: 250
- Protein: 3g
- Carbohydrates: 45g
- Fat: 6g
- Fiber: 3g

# Delicious Smoothie Recipes

## Strawberry Banana Smoothie with Almond Milk

*Introduction:* This classic smoothie combines the sweetness of strawberries with the creaminess of banana, blended together with almond milk for a refreshing and nutritious treat.
*Prep Time:* 5 minutes

*Ingredients:*
- 1 cup fresh or frozen strawberries
- 1 ripe banana
- 1 cup almond milk
- Optional: honey or maple syrup for added sweetness

*Instructions:*
1. Place strawberries, banana, and almond milk in a blender.
2. Blend until smooth and creamy.
3. Taste and add honey or maple syrup if desired.
4. Pour into glasses and serve immediately.
5. Enjoy this delightful strawberry banana smoothie with almond milk.

*Nutritional Information:* (per serving)
- Calories: 150
- Protein: 3g
- Carbohydrates: 30g
- Fat: 2g
- Fiber: 5g

## Spinach and Pineapple Smoothie with Coconut Water

*Introduction:* This vibrant green smoothie features nutrient-rich spinach and sweet pineapple, blended with hydrating coconut water for a refreshing and rejuvenating beverage.
*Prep Time:* 5 minutes

*Ingredients:*
- 2 cups fresh spinach leaves
- 1 cup fresh or frozen pineapple chunks

- 1 cup coconut water
- Optional: honey or agave syrup for added sweetness

*Instructions:*
1. Place spinach, pineapple chunks, and coconut water in a blender.
2. Blend until smooth and well combined.
3. Taste and add honey or agave syrup if desired.
4. Pour into glasses and serve immediately.
5. Enjoy this nutritious spinach and pineapple smoothie with coconut water.

*Nutritional Information:* (per serving)
- Calories: 120
- Protein: 2g
- Carbohydrates: 25g
- Fat: 1g
- Fiber: 4g

## Blueberry Kale Smoothie with Flaxseeds

*Introduction:* Packed with antioxidants and fiber, this blueberry kale smoothie with flaxseeds is a delicious way to boost your daily intake of nutrients and support overall health.
*Prep Time:* 5 minutes

*Ingredients:*
- 1 cup fresh or frozen blueberries
- 1 cup chopped kale leaves
- 1 tablespoon ground flaxseeds
- 1 cup almond milk or water
- Optional: honey or maple syrup for added sweetness

*Instructions:*
1. Combine blueberries, kale, flaxseeds, and almond milk (or water) in a blender.
2. Blend until smooth and creamy.
3. Taste and add honey or maple syrup if desired.
4. Blend again until well combined.
5. Pour into glasses and serve immediately.
6. Enjoy this nutritious blueberry kale smoothie with flaxseeds.

*Nutritional Information:* (per serving)
- Calories: 130
- Protein: 3g
- Carbohydrates: 20g
- Fat: 5g
- Fiber: 6g

# Mango Peach Smoothie with Greek Yogurt

*Introduction:* This creamy and tropical smoothie combines ripe mangoes and juicy peaches with creamy Greek yogurt for a delightful and satisfying beverage.
*Prep Time:* 5 minutes

*Ingredients:*
- 1 ripe mango, peeled and diced
- 1 ripe peach, pitted and diced
- 1/2 cup Greek yogurt
- 1/2 cup almond milk or water
- Optional: honey or agave syrup for added sweetness

*Instructions:*
1. Place diced mango, diced peach, Greek yogurt, and almond milk (or water) in a blender.
2. Blend until smooth and creamy.
3. Taste and add honey or agave syrup if desired.
4. Blend again until well combined.
5. Pour into glasses and serve immediately.
6. Enjoy this luscious mango peach smoothie with Greek yogurt.

*Nutritional Information:* (per serving)
- Calories: 150
- Protein: 6g
- Carbohydrates: 30g
- Fat: 2g
- Fiber: 4g

# Green Apple Smoothie with Spinach and Cucumber

*Introduction:* Crisp green apples, refreshing cucumber, and nutrient-packed spinach come together in this invigorating green smoothie, perfect for a revitalizing start to your day.
*Prep Time:* 5 minutes

*Ingredients:*
- 1 green apple, cored and chopped
- 1 cup fresh spinach leaves
- 1/2 cucumber, peeled and chopped
- 1/2 cup coconut water or water
- Optional: lemon juice and honey for added flavor

*Instructions:*
1. Combine chopped green apple, spinach leaves, cucumber, and coconut water (or water) in a blender.

2. Blend until smooth and well combined.
3. Add a splash of lemon juice and honey if desired, for extra flavor.
4. Blend again until thoroughly mixed.
5. Pour into glasses and serve immediately.
6. Enjoy this refreshing green apple smoothie with spinach and cucumber.

*Nutritional Information:* (per serving)
- Calories: 100
- Protein: 2g
- Carbohydrates: 25g
- Fat: 1g
- Fiber: 5g

## Pineapple Coconut Smoothie with Coconut Milk

*Introduction:* Transport yourself to a tropical paradise with this exotic pineapple coconut smoothie, featuring creamy coconut milk and sweet pineapple for a refreshing and indulgent treat.

*Prep Time:* 5 minutes

*Ingredients:*
- 1 cup fresh or frozen pineapple chunks
- 1/2 cup coconut milk
- 1/2 cup coconut water or water
- Optional: shredded coconut for garnish

*Instructions:*
1. Place pineapple chunks, coconut milk, and coconut water (or water) in a blender.
2. Blend until smooth and creamy.
3. Taste and adjust sweetness if necessary.
4. Pour into glasses and garnish with shredded coconut if desired.
5. Serve immediately and enjoy this tropical pineapple coconut smoothie.

*Nutritional Information:* (per serving)
- Calories: 150
- Protein: 1g
- Carbohydrates: 20g
- Fat: 8g
- Fiber: 3g

# Cherry Almond Smoothie with Chia Seeds

*Introduction:* This delightful cherry almond smoothie features the sweet tartness of cherries combined with the nutty flavor of almonds and the nutritional boost of chia seeds for a satisfying and nourishing beverage.
*Prep Time:* 5 minutes

*Ingredients:*
- 1 cup pitted cherries, fresh or frozen
- 1/4 cup almonds
- 1 tablespoon chia seeds
- 1 cup almond milk
- Optional: honey or maple syrup for added sweetness

*Instructions:*
1. Combine pitted cherries, almonds, chia seeds, and almond milk in a blender.
2. Blend until smooth and creamy.
3. Taste and add honey or maple syrup if desired.
4. Blend again until well combined.
5. Pour into glasses and serve immediately.
6. Enjoy this delicious cherry almond smoothie with chia seeds.

*Nutritional Information:* (per serving)
- Calories: 180
- Protein: 5g
- Carbohydrates: 25g
- Fat: 8g
- Fiber: 6g

# Orange Carrot Smoothie with Ginger

*Introduction:* Bright and invigorating, this orange carrot smoothie with ginger is bursting with vitamins and antioxidants, offering a refreshing and zesty start to your day.
*Prep Time:* 5 minutes

*Ingredients:*
- 2 oranges, peeled and segmented
- 1 large carrot, peeled and chopped
- 1-inch piece of fresh ginger, peeled
- 1/2 cup water or orange juice
- Optional: honey or agave syrup for added sweetness

*Instructions:*
1. Place orange segments, chopped carrot, peeled ginger, and water (or orange juice) in a blender.
2. Blend until smooth and well combined.
3. Taste and add honey or agave syrup if desired.
4. Blend again until thoroughly mixed.
5. Pour into glasses and serve immediately.
6. Enjoy this vibrant orange carrot smoothie with ginger.

*Nutritional Information:* (per serving)
- Calories: 100
- Protein: 2g
- Carbohydrates: 25g
- Fat: 1g
- Fiber: 5g

## Kiwi and Kale Smoothie with Coconut Water

*Introduction:* This energizing kiwi and kale smoothie with coconut water is bursting with vitamins and minerals, providing a refreshing and nutritious way to start your day or refuel after a workout.
*Prep Time:* 5 minutes

*Ingredients:*
- 2 kiwis, peeled and chopped
- 1 cup chopped kale leaves
- 1/2 cup coconut water
- 1/2 cup pineapple chunks (fresh or frozen)
- Optional: honey or agave syrup for added sweetness

*Instructions:*
1. Combine chopped kiwis, kale leaves, coconut water, and pineapple chunks in a blender.
2. Blend until smooth and creamy.
3. Taste and add honey or agave syrup if desired.
4. Blend again until well combined.
5. Pour into glasses and serve immediately.
6. Enjoy this revitalizing kiwi and kale smoothie with coconut water.

*Nutritional Information:* (per serving)
- Calories: 120
- Protein: 3g
- Carbohydrates: 25g
- Fat: 1g
- Fiber: 5g

## Mixed Berry Smoothie with Greek Yogurt

*Introduction:* Bursting with the flavors of mixed berries, this creamy smoothie features Greek yogurt for added protein and creaminess, making it a satisfying and nutritious choice for any time of day.
*Prep Time:* 5 minutes

*Ingredients:*
- 1 cup mixed berries (such as strawberries, blueberries, raspberries)
- 1/2 cup Greek yogurt
- 1/2 cup almond milk or water
- Optional: honey or agave syrup for added sweetness

*Instructions:*
1. Combine mixed berries, Greek yogurt, and almond milk (or water) in a blender.
2. Blend until smooth and well combined.
3. Taste and add honey or agave syrup if desired.
4. Blend again until thoroughly mixed.
5. Pour into glasses and serve immediately.
6. Enjoy this creamy mixed berry smoothie with Greek yogurt.

*Nutritional Information:* (per serving)
- Calories: 150
- Protein: 6g
- Carbohydrates: 25g
- Fat: 2g
- Fiber: 5g

## Avocado and Spinach Smoothie with Lime

*Introduction:* Creamy avocado and nutrient-rich spinach are blended with tangy lime juice in this invigorating smoothie, offering a burst of flavor and a boost of energy.
*Prep Time:* 5 minutes

*Ingredients:*
- 1 ripe avocado, peeled and pitted
- 1 cup fresh spinach leaves
- Juice of 1 lime
- 1 cup coconut water or water
- Optional: honey or agave syrup for added sweetness

*Instructions:*
1. Place peeled and pitted avocado, spinach leaves, lime juice, and coconut water (or water) in a blender.

2. Blend until smooth and creamy.
3. Taste and add honey or agave syrup if desired.
4. Blend again until well combined.
5. Pour into glasses and serve immediately.
6. Enjoy this refreshing avocado and spinach smoothie with lime.

*Nutritional Information:* (per serving)
- Calories: 200
- Protein: 3g
- Carbohydrates: 25g
- Fat: 10g
- Fiber: 8g

## Peach Raspberry Smoothie with Almond Milk

*Introduction:* Ripe peaches and tangy raspberries are blended with creamy almond milk in this delightful smoothie, offering a burst of summer flavors and plenty of nutrients.
*Prep Time:* 5 minutes

*Ingredients:*
- 1 ripe peach, peeled and diced
- 1/2 cup fresh or frozen raspberries
- 1 cup almond milk
- Optional: honey or agave syrup for added sweetness

*Instructions:*
1. Combine diced peach, raspberries, and almond milk in a blender.
2. Blend until smooth and creamy.
3. Taste and add honey or agave syrup if desired.
4. Blend again until thoroughly mixed.
5. Pour into glasses and serve immediately.
6. Enjoy this luscious peach raspberry smoothie with almond milk.

*Nutritional Information:* (per serving)
- Calories: 120
- Protein: 2g
- Carbohydrates: 20g
- Fat: 3g
- Fiber: 5g

## Watermelon Mint Smoothie with Lime

*Introduction:* Refreshing and hydrating, this watermelon mint smoothie with lime is the perfect summer drink, featuring juicy watermelon, fresh mint, and a splash of lime juice for a burst of flavor.
*Prep Time:* 5 minutes

*Ingredients:*
- 2 cups cubed watermelon
- 4-5 fresh mint leaves
- Juice of 1 lime
- 1/2 cup coconut water or water
- Optional: honey or agave syrup for added sweetness

*Instructions:*
1. Place cubed watermelon, mint leaves, lime juice, and coconut water (or water) in a blender.
2. Blend until smooth and well combined.
3. Taste and add honey or agave syrup if desired.
4. Blend again until thoroughly mixed.
5. Pour into glasses and serve immediately.
6. Enjoy this refreshing watermelon mint smoothie with lime.

*Nutritional Information:* (per serving)
- Calories: 80
- Protein: 1g
- Carbohydrates: 20g
- Fat: 1g
- Fiber: 2g

## Cucumber Celery Smoothie with Lemon

*Introduction:* Cool and revitalizing, this cucumber celery smoothie with lemon is packed with hydrating ingredients and zesty citrus flavor, making it the perfect pick-me-up on a hot day.
*Prep Time:* 5 minutes

*Ingredients:*
- 1 cucumber, peeled and chopped
- 2 celery stalks, chopped
- Juice of 1 lemon
- 1/2 cup coconut water or water
- Optional: honey or agave syrup for added sweetness

*Instructions:*
1. Combine chopped cucumber, celery stalks, lemon juice, and coconut water (or water) in a blender.
2. Blend until smooth and well combined.
3. Taste and add honey or agave syrup if desired.
4. Blend again until thoroughly mixed.
5. Pour into glasses and serve immediately.
6. Enjoy this cooling cucumber celery smoothie with lemon.

*Nutritional Information:* (per serving)
- Calories: 50
- Protein: 1g
- Carbohydrates: 15g
- Fat: 1g
- Fiber: 3g

## Papaya Mango Smoothie with Coconut Water

*Introduction:* Transport yourself to the tropics with this exotic papaya mango smoothie, featuring ripe papaya, sweet mango, and hydrating coconut water for a taste of paradise.
*Prep Time:* 5 minutes

*Ingredients:*
- 1 cup diced papaya
- 1 cup diced mango
- 1/2 cup coconut water
- 1/2 cup pineapple chunks (fresh or frozen)
- Optional: honey or agave syrup for added sweetness

*Instructions:*
1. Place diced papaya, diced mango, coconut water, and pineapple chunks in a blender.
2. Blend until smooth and creamy.
3. Taste and add honey or agave syrup if desired.
4. Blend again until well combined.
5. Pour into glasses and serve immediately.
6. Enjoy this tropical papaya mango smoothie with coconut water.

*Nutritional Information:* (per serving)
- Calories: 140
- Protein: 2g
- Carbohydrates: 30g
- Fat: 1g
- Fiber: 5g

# 30-Day Meal Plan

**Week 1:**

**Day 1:**
- **Breakfast:** Pg 42 - Apple Cinnamon Overnight Oats
- **Lunch:** Pg 49 - Turkey and Avocado Wrap with Lettuce and Tomato
- **Dinner:** Pg 60 - Baked Salmon with Lemon and Dill

**Day 2:**
- **Breakfast:** Pg 47 - Green Smoothie with Kale, Pineapple, and Ginger
- **Lunch:** Pg 53 - Greek Chickpea Salad with Feta and Olives
- **Dinner:** Pg 61 - Turkey Chili with Kidney Beans and Bell Peppers

**Day 3:**
- **Breakfast:** Pg 40 - Quinoa Breakfast Bowl with Almond Milk and Fruit
- **Lunch:** Pg 51 - Spinach Salad with Grilled Chicken and Balsamic Dressing
- **Dinner:** Pg 61 - Grilled Chicken Breast with Roasted Vegetables

**Day 4:**
- **Breakfast:** Pg 45 - Peanut Butter Banana Smoothie with Flaxseed
- **Lunch:** Pg 52 - Cauliflower Rice Bowl with Black Beans and Avocado
- **Dinner:** Pg 62 - Quinoa Stuffed Bell Peppers with Tomato Sauce

**Day 5:**
- **Breakfast:** Pg 41 - Whole Grain Toast with Almond Butter and Sliced Banana
- **Lunch:** Pg 54 - Turkey Meatballs with Zucchini Noodles and Marinara Sauce
- **Dinner:** Pg 63 - Shrimp Stir-Fry with Broccoli and Snow Peas

**Day 6:**
- **Breakfast:** Pg 44 - Smoothie Bowl with Mixed Berries and Granola
- **Lunch:** Pg 55 - Roasted Vegetable and Quinoa Bowl with Tahini Dressing
- **Dinner:** Pg 64 - Baked Cod with Herbed Quinoa

**Day 7:**
- **Breakfast:** Pg 46 - Almond Flour Waffles with Fresh Berries
- **Lunch:** Pg 56 - Egg Salad Lettuce Wraps with Dill
- **Dinner:** Pg 65 - Veggie and Lentil Curry with Brown Rice

**Week 2:**

**Day 8:**
- **Breakfast:** Pg 43 - Veggie Omelette with Goat Cheese
- **Lunch:** Pg 57 - Tomato Basil Soup with Whole Grain Crackers

- **Dinner:** Pg 66 - Zucchini Noodles with Tomato Basil Sauce

**Day 9:**
- **Breakfast:** Pg 44 - Chia Seed Pudding with Mango and Coconut
- **Lunch:** Pg 58 - Sushi Bowl with Brown Rice, Avocado, and Cucumber
- **Dinner:** Pg 67 - Lemon Garlic Roasted Chicken with Steamed Green Beans

**Day 10:**
- **Breakfast:** Pg 47 - Green Smoothie with Kale, Pineapple, and Ginger
- **Lunch:** Pg 59 - Turkey and Quinoa Stuffed Peppers
- **Dinner:** Pg 68 - Turkey and Vegetable Skewers with Quinoa Pilaf

**Day 11:**
- **Breakfast:** Pg 42 - Apple Cinnamon Overnight Oats
- **Lunch:** Pg 61 - Chicken and Vegetable Stir-Fry with Brown Rice
- **Dinner:** Pg 69 - Stuffed Portobello Mushrooms with Spinach and Goat Cheese

**Day 12:**
- **Breakfast:** Pg 45 - Peanut Butter Banana Smoothie with Flaxseed
- **Lunch:** Pg 57 - Sweet Potato and Black Bean Quesadilla with Salsa
- **Dinner:** Pg 70 - Roasted Butternut Squash and Chickpea Salad

**Day 13:**
- **Breakfast:** Pg 46 - Almond Flour Waffles with Fresh Berries
- **Lunch:** Pg 71 - Veggie Stir-Fry with Tofu and Brown Rice
- **Dinner:** Pg 71 - Baked Chicken Thighs with Sweet Potatoes and Brussels Sprouts

**Day 14:**
- **Breakfast:** Pg 41 - Muesli with Yogurt and Sliced Peaches
- **Lunch:** Pg 57 - Tomato Basil Soup with Whole Grain Crackers
- **Dinner:** Pg 72 - Spaghetti Squash with Garlic and Parmesan

**Week 3:**

**Day 15:**
- **Breakfast:** Pg 43 - Veggie Omelette with Goat Cheese
- **Lunch:** Pg 58 - Sushi Bowl with Brown Rice, Avocado, and Cucumber
- **Dinner:** Pg 60 - Baked Salmon with Lemon and Dill

**Day 16:**
- **Breakfast:** Pg 42 - Apple Cinnamon Overnight Oats
- **Lunch:** Pg 59 - Turkey and Quinoa Stuffed Peppers
- **Dinner:** Pg 61 - Chicken and Vegetable Stir-Fry with Brown Rice

**Day 17:**
- **Breakfast:** Pg 47 - Green Smoothie with Kale, Pineapple, and Ginger
- **Lunch:** Pg 61 - Turkey Chili with Kidney Beans and Bell Peppers
- **Dinner:** Pg 62 - Quinoa Stuffed Bell Peppers with Tomato Sauce

**Day 18:**
- **Breakfast:** Pg 44 - Chia Seed Pudding with Mango and Coconut
- **Lunch:** Pg 53 - Greek Chickpea Salad with Feta and Olives
- **Dinner:** Pg 63 - Shrimp Stir-Fry with Broccoli and Snow Peas

**Day 19:**
- **Breakfast:** Pg 46 - Almond Flour Waffles with Fresh Berries
- **Lunch:** Pg 57 - Sweet Potato and Black Bean Quesadilla with Salsa
- **Dinner:** Pg 64 - Baked Cod with Herbed Quinoa

**Day 20:**
- **Breakfast:** Pg 41 - Muesli with Yogurt and Sliced Peaches
- **Lunch:** Pg 52 - Cauliflower Rice Bowl with Black Beans and Avocado
- **Dinner:** Pg 65 - Veggie and Lentil Curry with Brown Rice

**Day 21:**
- **Breakfast:** Pg 43 - Veggie Omelette with Goat Cheese
- **Lunch:** Pg 58 - Sushi Bowl with Brown Rice, Avocado, and Cucumber
- **Dinner:** Pg 66 - Zucchini Noodles with Tomato Basil Sauce

**Week 4:**

**Day 22:**
- **Breakfast:** Pg 42 - Apple Cinnamon Overnight Oats
- **Lunch:** Pg 53 - Greek Chickpea Salad with Feta and Olives
- **Dinner:** Pg 67 - Lemon Garlic Roasted Chicken with Steamed Green Beans

**Day 23:**
- **Breakfast:** Pg 44 - Chia Seed Pudding with Mango and Coconut
- **Lunch:** Pg 54 - Turkey Meatballs with Zucchini Noodles and Marinara Sauce
- **Dinner:** Pg 68 - Turkey and Vegetable Skewers with Quinoa Pilaf

**Day 24:**
- **Breakfast:** Pg 46 - Almond Flour Waffles with Fresh Berries
- **Lunch:** Pg 55 - Roasted Vegetable and Quinoa Bowl with Tahini Dressing
- **Dinner:** Pg 69 - Stuffed Portobello Mushrooms with Spinach and Goat Cheese

**Day 25:**
- **Breakfast:** Pg 47 - Green Smoothie with Kale, Pineapple, and Ginger

- **Lunch:** Pg 56 - Egg Salad Lettuce Wraps with Dill
- **Dinner:** Pg 70 - Roasted Butternut Squash and Chickpea Salad

**Day 26:**
- **Breakfast:** Pg 41 - Muesli with Yogurt and Sliced Peaches
- **Lunch:** Pg 57 - Sweet Potato and Black Bean Quesadilla with Salsa
- **Dinner:** Pg 71 - Veggie Stir-Fry with Tofu and Brown Rice

**Day 27:**
- **Breakfast:** Pg 43 - Veggie Omelette with Goat Cheese
- **Lunch:** Pg 58 - Sushi Bowl with Brown Rice, Avocado, and Cucumber
- **Dinner:** Pg 71 - Baked Chicken Thighs with Sweet Potatoes and Brussels Sprouts

**Day 28:**
- **Breakfast:** Pg 42 - Apple Cinnamon Overnight Oats
- **Lunch:** Pg 57 - Tomato Basil Soup with Whole Grain Crackers
- **Dinner:** Pg 72 - Spaghetti Squash with Garlic and Parmesan

**Week 5:**

**Day 29:**
- **Breakfast:** Pg 43 - Veggie Omelette with Goat Cheese
- **Lunch:** Pg 58 - Sushi Bowl with Brown Rice, Avocado, and Cucumber
- **Dinner:** Pg 60 - Baked Salmon with Lemon and Dill

**Day 30:**
- **Breakfast:** Pg 42 - Apple Cinnamon Overnight Oats
- **Lunch:** Pg 59 - Turkey and Quinoa Stuffed Peppers
- **Dinner:** Pg 61 - Chicken and Vegetable Stir-Fry with Brown Rice

## Note to Readers:

This 30-Day Meal Plan provides a diverse range of recipes carefully selected to support individuals managing acid reflux. It emphasizes whole, nutrient-rich foods while minimizing triggers that can exacerbate symptoms.

Feel free to adjust the meal plan based on your preferences and dietary needs. Remember to stay hydrated throughout the day and listen to your body's cues. Incorporating regular physical activity and practicing mindful eating can further enhance your overall well-being.

# Premium Bonuses for Maximum Benefits of this Cookbook

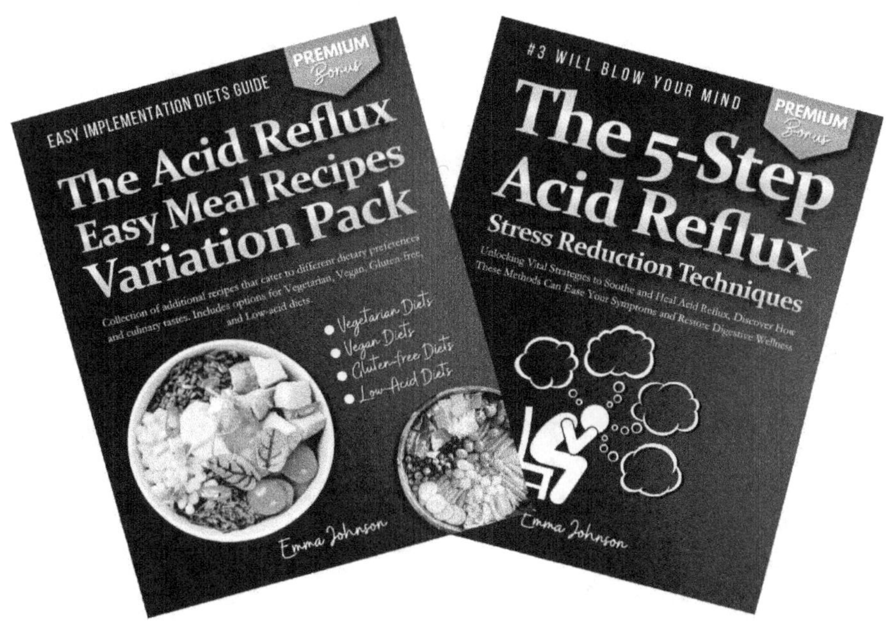

To Download The 5-Step Acid Reflux, go to:
https://tinyurl.com/5stepreflux
Or scan QR CODE below:

To Download The Acid Reflux Easy Meal Recipes Variation Pack, go to:
https://tinyurl.com/acidpack
Or scan QR CODE below:

9 798324 566906